COLLAB   TIVE

Interprofessi
Interpersona

SECOND EDITION

SALLY HORNBY & JO ATKINS

With contributions from

HILARY BEALE
MARGARET CAMPBELL
LARRY SANDERS

b

**Blackwell
Science**

© 1993, 2000 by
Blackwell Science Ltd
Editorial Offices:
Osney Mead, Oxford OX2 0EL
25 John Street, London WC1N 2BS
23 Ainslie Place, Edinburgh EH3 6AJ
350 Main Street, Malden
   MA 02148 5018, USA
54 University Street, Carlton
   Victoria 3053, Australia
10, rue Casimir Delavigne
   75006 Paris, France

Other Editorial Offices:

Blackwell Wissenschafts-Verlag GmbH
Kurfürstendamm 57
10707 Berlin, Germany

Blackwell Science KK
MG Kodenmacho Building
7–10 Kodenmacho Nihombashi
Chuo-ku, Tokyo 104, Japan

The right of the Author to be identified as the
Author of this Work has been asserted in
accordance with the Copyright, Designs and
Patents Act 1988.

First Edition published 1993, Second Edition
published 2000

Set in 10/12pt Souvenir
by DP Photosetting, Aylesbury, Bucks
Printed and bound in Great Britain by
Alden Press, Oxford

Marston Book Services Ltd
PO Box 269
Abingdon
Oxon OX14 4YN
(Orders: Tel: 01235 465500
           Fax: 01235 465555)

USA
Blackwell Science, Inc.
Commerce Place
350 Main Street
Malden, MA 02148 5018
(Orders: Tel: 800 759 6102
                781 388 8250
           Fax: 781 388 8255

Canada
Login Brothers Book Company
324 Saulteaux Crescent
Winnipeg, Manitoba R3J 3T2
(Orders: Tel: 204 837–2987
           Fax: 204 837-3116)

Australia
Blackwell Science Pty Ltd
54 University Street
Carlton, Victoria 3053
(Orders: Tel: 03 9347 0300
           Fax: 03 9347 5001)

A catalogue record for this title is available
from the British Library

ISBN 0-632-05669-X

Library of Congress
Cataloging-in-Publication Data
is available

For further information on
Blackwell Science, visit our website:
www.blackwell-science.com

Contents

List of Examples

Preface to the Second Edition

For the First Edition of *Collaborative Care: interprofessional, interagency and interpersonal*, Sally Hornby, at the age of 83, wrote a personal, reflective and retrospective account of her professional life as a psychotherapist and social work practitioner in west London in the 1950s through to the 1980s. She used her extensive observations, experience and training to consider issues of collaboration and the complexities of relationships between clients and faceworkers, faceworkers and agencies, and agencies and professional groups. Her emphasis was on the nature of human relations rather than the structural or organisational issues that are more often the subject of press releases and inquiries when failures occur. Sally Hornby's aim was to provide insights and understandings into the complexities of collaborative relationships so that individuals and groups could take constructive action to identify hindrances and attempt to overcome them.

The pioneering work of Sally Hornby into the complex and subtle nature of collaboration in health and social care has been retained and expanded in the Second Edition. The team that came together in 1999 to work with Sally to develop the themes of the book found themselves in agreement both with the aims of collaborative working at the client/user interface and with the need for an update and review of the relational approach she advocated. The team considered that if the aim of collaborative care is to provide optimal levels of care then not only the transboundary relationships between individual faceworkers and agencies needed to be addressed but also transboundary relationships between faceworkers and the managers or planners of services in their organisations. The relational approach advocated by Sally Hornby encourages enhanced dialogue and non-defensive, open approach to participative planning. By attending to these aspects of collaboration the team hoped to address the added complexities that can arise from the political, economic and organisational contexts of modern service delivery.

The framework adopted by Sally in the First Edition identified hindrances to collaboration with the intention of providing a greater understanding, awareness and constructive action towards them on the part of faceworkers at ground level. Using both psychodynamic and systems theories Sally explored the concept of boundary, the psychodynamics of groups, the defensive behaviours of individuals, groups and organisations and their coping mechanisms, in an attempt to provide insights into relational aspects of collaboration.

The additional material that makes up the new Part III, (Organisations and Contexts), maintains this focus and draws upon the same theoretical ideas to expand the concepts into an exploration of the effects of environmental influences on faceworkers and professional groups working at the ground level. Key issues such as the fight for resources, the tendency of professionals to behave defensively towards their clients, departments and resources, and the use of individual and group coping mechanisms are revisited. The new focus adds reflections on the effects of professional and organisational contexts on these issues and provides new perspectives on the effectiveness of helping relationships in the year 2000 and beyond.

The case-study style of the first edition has been retained by the team, with examples being drawn from personal experiences, interviews with colleagues and members of the Carers Forum, case conferences, recent legal cases and relevant literature. The work draws on the themes of Sally Hornby's original text and her psychodynamic and systems framework. As with Sally's original work the additional material has been planned with particular reference to faceworkers. The aim of the material in Part III is to provide understanding and insight into the nature of organisational influences on the work of helpers and carers. It is hoped that these new perspectives will enable faceworkers to extend their helping relationships by working constructively and collaboratively with the senior staff and managers in their own organisations.

Throughout this new third section the contributors have striven to maintain the flavour and style of the first two sections in order to produce a cohesive text based on the experience of a reflective, psychodynamic practitioner. Though the first-person reflective stance taken by Sally Hornby could not be duplicated the team have used a very similar approach, drawing on themes and issues from the case studies and recent experiences in their own practices. Shared learning across the group, under the leadership of Sally Hornby, has led to new perspectives on the nature of anxiety-driven practices and ways of overcoming negative consequences in the interest of achieving satisfying, effective, collaborative, ground level, faceworker-client relationships.

The new work has been developed by Sally herself, three members of staff from Oxford Brookes University, and Larry Sanders, Legal Advisor to the Carers' Forum and Community Care Rights Advisor for Oxfordshire. Hilary Beale is a Multiprofessional Course Co-ordinator in the School of Social Sciences and Law at the University. Margaret Campbell is a Senior Lecturer and experienced practitioner in psychodynamics and psychotherapy in the School of Health Care. Jo Atkins was a Principal Lecturer at the University until 1999, and is now a consultant on current systems thinking in a variety of organisations.

Sadly, Sally Hornby died on 28 December 1999 before the final draft for the new edition was completed. Although Sally is not with us to share in the new publication, the team takes comfort from being certain that she was very excited to know that her work would be revised for the Second Edition. All members of the team feel that it was a great privilege to have worked so closely with such an inspiring lady.

Jo Atkins
Oxford
March 2000

Foreword

When Sally Hornby first published this book it was not too difficult a task to write the foreword. We wrote then that her book was not only 'timely but necessary'. We referred to a seemingly endless set of acronyms: E.M.P.E (European network for multiprofessional education); C.A.I.P.E (Centre for the advancement of Interprofessional Education); M.C.T (Marylebone Centre Trust); J.I.P.C (Journal of Interprofessional Care); C.O.N.C.A.H (Continuing Care at Home); C.I.P.S (Centre for Interprofessional Studies).

Today we would need to add a further twenty, and Janet Storrie's (1992) survey of higher education courses in multiprofessional studies would number over 100 and not fifteen as it did then.

Sally, who sadly passed away last year, has left us a worthy foundation to all the developments that have taken place. Her work, because of its detailed and minutely described observations on the nature and difficulties of multi-professional work, should now become even more sought-after as report after report repeats the need for partnership/collaboration/shared work/reflective practice, within health and social care agencies.

It is for this reason that Sally Hornby's co-author, Jo Atkins, and her colleagues have added a much-needed section on organisations and context. As we experience a never-ending series of 're-organisations' between primary care groups and trusts, regional offices and health authorities, social service and local authority boundaries, the requirement to understand and separate the individual and institutional anxieties engendered is yet again 'timely and necessary'. 'Overcoming defensive behaviour', a section in this new Part III, will become an essential survival pamphlet for all health and social care practitioners.

We write this foreword having received on our desks the national plan for the future of our health service. It is a tribute to all involved with this edition, but especially to Sally Hornby, that if this national plan is to be implemented in any meaningful way, then the contents of this book could easily serve as the managers'/teachers' guide to its future implementation.

Marilyn J Pietroni and Patrick C Pietroni
Dept of Postgraduate General Practice
T.P.M.D.E. London University

Acknowledgements

I wish first to acknowledge the debt I owe to all the people – users, informal and formal carers, practitioners of many professions – with whom, over the years, I have gained experience and understanding, discussed practice and ideas. In particular I appreciate the help of all those with whom I worked on the problems of collaboration, in the 1970s and 1980s in Paddington, Kensington and Chelsea. Without their collaboration the material for this book would not have been available. They are too many to name, but I must single out two for special thanks – Jane Coleridge, at the time director of Kensington & Chelsea MIND, and Dr Richard Stone, a GP in the area. I also wish to thank Isabel Menzies Lyth, who helped me understand the psychodynamic aspects of collaborative problems; David Millard and Patrick Pietroni, who encouraged me to write and publish; Elizabeth Ratiu, Win Roberts and Bob Morley for their support throughout. Finally, my thanks go to Lisa Field and Caroline Savage, for all their goodwill, patience and help in publishing.

For funding some of my work, I owe a debt of gratitude to the Lord Ashdown Trust.

Acknowledgements to Second Edition

All the contributors to this Second Edition wish to express their appreciation of the work of the Oxfordshire Carers' Forum and the many 'faceworkers' whose experiences have helped to shape the focus and content of this new book.

Part I
Collaboration

Chapter 1
Introduction

Many people involved in the helping services see the need for collaboration with other helpers but find that it is not always easy. I write this book for them: carers, practitioners of all the helping professions, workers with varying levels of training, and self-helpers. The common denominator of this large and disparate set of people is their inevitable involvement in certain kinds of personal and group relationships which, to a greater or lesser extent, are determined by their helping role. These relationships have much in common, whatever the context in which help is offered or the particular skills required.

During recent years reports have repeatedly emphasised the importance of collaboration in order to provide optimal care. The problems of improving and co-ordinating services have been tackled in many different ways and at all levels of service provision: through joint planning, major restructuring of services, development of models for primary health care, joint projects, refinement of procedures, production of guidelines, and not least through the co-operative efforts of workers at ground level. Despite these developments there are still innumerable examples of failure in collaboration. A few attract publicity but many more go unnoticed except by those involved, who are aware that the help provided could have been better.

At the point of delivery services have to be combined and individualised; and if needs are to be met adequately it is crucial that people working together at this level relate well with each other. A structural approach to collaborative problems must therefore be paralleled by a relational approach – that is, one which is concerned with the human element in working together.

If help can be provided from a single agency or within one department of a large agency, working relationships can develop over time, in teams or other groups, supported by agency structures. Although there may be collaborative problems between workers of various professions and training, these are not compounded by the need to work across the agency or departmental boundary. Frequently, however, help is needed from more than one agency and has to be specifically put together to meet a particular situation, each one requiring a slightly different combination of services, workers and skills. For those who work under these conditions, the inescapable conclusion is that the intention to collaborate does not in itself bring about the desired result; goodwill is not enough.

I first became aware of just how difficult collaboration across professional and agency boundaries could be and what demands it makes on workers, when I was organising a course on psychotherapeutic skills and their integration into the practice of various professions. The course was provided by practitioners in an NHS centre for psychotherapy. They were aware that much psychotherapeutic work was already being carried out with people who would never cross the threshold of the centre; so it seemed a good use of time to help workers in other agencies to develop their psychotherapeutic skills and, at the same time, facilitate a better use of the specialist psychotherapy service, through improving working relations with the surrounding agencies. The course catered for about 50 people – health, social and voluntary agency workers, teachers, clergymen, policemen and other experienced workers. Because it was only open to those working in the locality many of the participants already knew and worked with each other. The course took an afternoon a week for 30 weeks. The programme was carried out in small and large groups which were loosely structured but task-orientated – the small groups on such themes as working with individuals, families, adolescents, the large group on the general theme of the integration of psychotherapeutic work with other forms of help.

After a while considerable trust was built up between participants and frequently the discussion turned from the worker's relationship with the person in need of help to relationships between workers themselves. Here, despite the wish to integrate their various forms of help, it seemed that collaboration often proved unexpectedly difficult. In one large group meeting the following exchange took place:

The opening scene

A group of about 30 practitioners, from various professions and agencies in a particular inner-city locality, are in the middle of a discussion on the difficulties of helping disorganised families with multiple problems.

TEACHER: When the parents of my pupils are being helped by other people, I find it odd that so often they don't make contact with me. Why don't they?

HEALTH VISITOR: When you speak about 'my pupils and their parents', I keep on thinking 'these are my families'.

SOCIAL WORKER: And they are my clients.

GP: (half jokingly but with feeling) Not to be outdone, I must establish that they are my patients.

AREA SOCIAL WORKER: I get angry with hospital social workers who often use the word 'patient' when they are talking with doctors. Why don't they say 'client'? After all they are social workers.

HOSPITAL SOCIAL WORKER: Sometimes I feel I'm more in tune with doctors than I am with area social workers.

TEACHER: We were discussing disorganised families not disorganised social workers! What I wanted to know was, who should take responsibility for contacting other workers.

The discussion came back to the question.

This opening scene points to various problems affecting collaboration: the divisiveness of language, professional possessiveness, professional identity, and the issue of responsibility for initiating contact with other workers. In further exchanges it became evident that these problems overlaid other relational difficulties that were less obvious.

From discussions on this course I realised that if workers could collaborate better the help offered would be considerably improved without the need for any extra provision. To achieve this a greater understanding of the nature of working relationships across professional, agency and other boundaries was needed. Only then would it become clearer what knowledge, ability and changes in attitude would be required of workers, and what part the professions and agencies would need to play in enabling workers to develop and exercise collaborative skills. Since then I have tried to identify and study the hindrances to collaboration which result from transboundary relationships between helpers, drawing on my experience of working in a variety of interprofessional and interagency situations.

Collaboration is important at all levels but I am here concerned with help at ground, or delivery, level. This is not to diminish the importance of collaboration at other levels; it is a matter of focusing on a particular aspect of a large subject, and writing only from personal experience. Thus I do not contribute directly to discussions concerning the failures in collaboration which have led to inquiries, nor to the particular problems of ethnic or other minority groups. However, although the material presented in this book is limited to my particular experience, the resulting understanding concerning common hindrances to collaboration can be directly applied to innumerable other situations. I do not attempt to give blueprints for collaboration, human relationships being too complex; it is through increased understanding and awareness that people are enabled to improve their relational skills. If common patterns of difficulty in working relationships are identified, described and named, it becomes easier for workers to spot them early and take measures to deal with them sooner rather than later. My aim is to further understanding in such a way that workers themselves turn it to practical use.

This is therefore a practical book and I introduce very little specific theory. However, it is necessary to have a conceptual framework within which to discuss collaborative relationships, and for this I have drawn on systems theory and psychodynamic theories. They have helped me to understand and formulate my experiences of collaborative work, and to order my thoughts about the processes which occur in working relationships across important personal and group boundaries. I give no references in the text, but a list of books for further reading is provided.

In the first part of the book, I use a relational approach to look at collaboration. I start with examples of common hindrances, and explore their causes; then, illustrate and discuss essential elements of effective collaborative practice. In the second part, I put forward a way of looking at helping relationships that is based on the fundamental human need for a secure and satisfying identity, in the achievement of which working roles play a significant part. From this it is possible to suggest ways of reducing the problems and indicate lines of development for improving collaborative practice. The suggestions are tentative and designed to open up the subject rather than give definitive answers.

Key concepts

Before embarking on examples of collaborative difficulties, I need to explain a few key concepts and terms.

Boundary
The defining limit of any system; in human terms, of any person or group of people or organisation. All workers function within some group boundary, that of agency, profession, family, neighbourhood or some other kind. These boundaries, whilst essential to optimal help, do, at the same time, impede it. They are essential for the provision of specialised services and skills; but they also create hindrances to the co-ordination and integration of these same services and skills, when more than one is needed.

Boundaries delineate identity and also set limits. They are needed by professions, agencies and individual workers to define what they do and to set limits to what they are expected to do, whether by the user of their services, other workers or themselves. Collaboration requires working at the interface of a number of different boundaries: those between individuals – helper and the one needing help, personal carer and worker, fellow workers; and those between organised groups – professions, agencies, community groups. Problems seem to be inherent in human relationships, not only at the personal interface but also when relating across group boundaries. The boundaries of professions and agencies are often strongly maintained, and it is for this reason that, although much of this book applies to all helpers, certain parts focus solely on professional practitioners and the formal agencies. It is essential to tackle the problems of relations between these powerful organisations and institutions at managerial levels but this approach by itself can never achieve an effective solution to collaborative problems at ground level, where the individual person – whether helper or helped – is so important.

Boundary overlap
The shared area in which helping tasks may be carried out, for instance by personal carer, care-workers and practitioners, or by one or another practitioner. Overlap areas are of particular importance to collaboration: on the positive side they provide flexibility; on the negative, they may engender uncertainty, mistrust and rivalry.

Identity
The sense of being someone, the uniqueness of an individual or a group. Group identity derives from certain factors which are held in common by those in the group. Individual identity is built up from a number of different sources: personality; identification with family, cultural, racial groups, etc.; the assumption of particular roles – gender, social, professional, etc. The fact that individual identity is often enhanced by the working role may influence a person's attitudes and behaviour in a collaborative situation.

The basic caring relationship
The human relationship that should always exist, however minimally, between those in the roles of helper and helped. Its essential characteristics are concern and respect for the individual. The nature of helping relationships varies very considerably from one situation to another but, though modified by the different roles that helpers fill, the relationship always retains certain essential characteristics. The basic relationship is the same for all those involved in helping, from the most highly to the least skilled. It is the identifying factor which they all share.

Collaboration
A relationship between two or more people, groups or organisations working together to define and achieve a common purpose. At delivery level, collaboration takes place between the people who need some kind of help and the people who provide it, and between the providers. Its importance varies from one helping situation to another, but it can be a key element in many methods of help, whether medical, social or psychological.

Terminology

In addressing this book to all those involved in a helping role at ground level I try to use basic English but have found it necessary to use special terms to embody concepts relating to collaboration. This vocabulary is designed to be useful when communicating about shared areas of work. In the opening scene the lack of a common language was immediately apparent. My aim has been to find a vocabulary acceptable to all those working at ground level.

User
People in need of help are at present defined either in terms of the person

who is offering it – as 'patient' or 'client' – or of the setting in which help is offered – as 'resident' or 'member'. These definitions of the one using help are all valid within their own context, but they are limiting and inappropriate to a context in which transboundary collaboration is needed. I have settled for the word 'user' to describe the individual, couple, family or other group which uses help. This collective term serves to emphasise an important underlying value; those who use help are now defined in their own terms, not in terms of the profession or agency providing help. There is a reorientation: instead of putting the helper or agency in the centre of the picture, pride of place is given to the user, who is then less likely to be put in an inferior position by the helpers, or fragmented by their specialisms.

Faceworker
Having settled on the term 'user', what then should be the corresponding word to cover all those who are helping the user at ground level as distinct from managerial levels? From the user's viewing-point, these workers are the human face of the helping services, the faces that are known. As helpers they all work at the interface with users, so I think of them as 'faceworkers'. There are probably more helpers outside the formal helping services than in them – family, friends, neighbours and others in the local community – who are also faceworkers. However much the help they offer may differ, all those who work directly with users have something in common: the facework relationship.

Trouble
The third comprehensive term that I find essential from the beginning is one to describe all the things that may bring a user to seek help. I have adopted the word 'trouble'. Problems, illness, disability, dependency, disadvantage and maladjustment in the spheres of material, physical, emotional, mental, personal and social life, may all be experienced as troubles by the user. And, wherever help is sought, it can come naturally to ask: 'What is the trouble?' Again, the word supports an approach to helping which does not fragment the user.

In introducing these terms, there is no intention to supplant professional terminologies, which serve essential purposes; however, they are not always adequate when talking about collaborative practice. In the following chapters I introduce further new terms and redefine old ones, in order to build a basic collaborative vocabulary. A glossary is given at the end of the book. The use of such a terminology and some of the words themselves may at first seem strange, unnecessary and tiresome. Having found them essential for clarifying collaborative concepts, I make no apology for their use, but I wish to forewarn readers. The terminology has simplified my task of communicating simultaneously to all faceworkers, but only if a word should prove itself useful in everyday working life, will it find its way into common usage.

I have also used language in the service of a particular approach to helping. The way in which thoughts are ordered is influenced by, and in turn influences, thinking and communication. I hope therefore that the framework and vocabulary which I adopt in the following chapters will contribute to the development of an effective collaborative approach to helping – one which, whilst recognising and valuing essential differences, seeks to establish the common ground in all helping relationships.

I have found it impossible to write about collaboration without incorporating certain values. These have led to a user-centred model, in contrast to a practitioner or agency-centred one. It is illustrated in diagramatic form in Fig. 1.1. Readers may not entirely agree with my approach; similarly, faceworkers when collaborating may not start from the same value base as each other. This is inevitable, and recognition of such differences is often an important factor in successful collaboration.

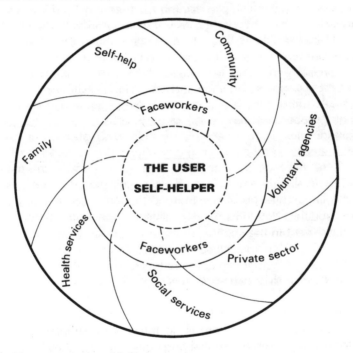

Fig. 1.1   The user-centred model of help.

Chapter 2
Difficulties in Working Together

It may only be when difficulties become serious that lack of collaboration is considered as a possible cause. Often the seeds of collaborative failure lie deep and may have gone unnoticed for a long time. Making and maintaining the collaborative relationships necessary for optimal help takes time and effort and, since all faceworkers are busy, collaboration is often overlooked or shelved, until problems begin to arise as a result of its absence. It also requires awareness and skill. In this chapter I give seven cases illustrating collaborative problems and from them demonstrate common underlying causes. If the examples also show lack of skill in practitioners, this is in no way to single out a particular profession; every faceworker knows that at times their collaboration has been less than perfect.

I take examples from quite ordinary helping situations, not wishing to focus on the case so much as on the relational processes which it demonstrates. Some have been taken from past years, and circumstances may have changed slightly since then. This is unimportant, since the cases describe collaborative problems that occur frequently in many different situations, and the relational processes illustrated are likely to apply to a wide variety of working situations.

Mrs Anson, the day nursery mother

A single parent family, consisting of the mother, Mrs Anson and three children, was known to the health visitor as a disorganised family, with a mother who did not function very well but had considerable warmth for her children. The health visitor had a supportive relationship with Mrs Anson and the family did not stand out from many similar ones on her caseload. It was when the eldest child started school that attention became focused on this family. The little girl often arrived late, dishevelled and sometimes dirty. The education welfare officer visited the home and alerted the social services department, saying that he had found the mother drunk and shouting at the children, and he felt her care of them was inadequate. When the social worker visited, she thought Mrs Anson seemed depressed and not coping well. She contacted the health visitor, and they agreed that Mrs Anson should have social work help

10

and the younger children be found places in a day nursery. The mother fell in with these plans. There was initial contact between the social worker and the head of the day nursery; this was not maintained, but the health visitor made a link between them.

The day nursery staff were worried because Mrs Anson often brought the children late. There was a rule that children who were not in the nursery by 11 AM could not be given lunch. The staff found themselves breaking the rule for these children and, in order to avoid this, one of them who passed the family's door in the morning started picking up the children. Sometimes they were bathed at the nursery and their clothes washed. The staff became very attached to the children and liked the mother, whom they found a 'poor thing' but fond of the children and always appreciative of what was done for them.

Mrs Anson gradually became more demanding of help from the social worker who, having begun by responding, then felt it time to call a halt, judging her to be capable of coping more independently. She therefore started to encourage Mrs Anson to do more for herself and tried to help her become better organised in managing her money and running her home. This change of policy was mentioned to the health visitor but not to the nursery staff.

From a casual conversation in the nursery, the health visitor heard about the special help the children were getting and also heard the nursery nurses criticising the social worker for being too hard with the mother and not giving her enough support. The health visitor agreed with the social worker's aims and explained them to the nursery nurses but felt that they remained unconvinced. In the ensuing discussion, they expressed criticism of social workers generally, for not being firmer with some other mothers, but they felt sorry for Mrs Anson. The health visitor discussed the situation with the social worker who was angry with the nursery staff, saying they were undermining her help. It was agreed that a meeting would be useful.

This was attended by the headmistress, class teacher and education welfare officer, the head of the nursery and two nursery nurses (as the children were in different groups), the health visitor, the social worker and her senior who chaired the meeting. It was soon apparent that the school workers, social workers and health visitor were in agreement on the joint line to be taken. The headmistress said that now she had met the social worker face-to-face and heard about her relationship with Mrs Anson, she felt she could be firmer with the latter and expect a little more from her. The nursery head was less committed to this line, realising that her staff were not going along with it and she continued to discuss the question of how much could be expected of Mrs Anson. The social worker gave some instances of the way the latter had changed recently. The nursery head then questioned whether, if this were so, it had been right to place both younger children in the day nursery. The social worker defended her action, spoke at length about the need to develop a good working relationship, and how perhaps nursery nurses did not fully appreciate the importance of this. She had needed to build up such a relationship with the mother before becoming firmer, as part of a planned process. The health visitor, who appreciated the nursery nurses' position, queried this. The social worker had to agree that her method had not been planned in advance and that perhaps she had acted rather precipitately at the beginning. She also apologised for not having kept in closer touch with the nursery and not having explained the changes in her method of help. The nursery head turned to her staff and discussed with them the significance of the social worker's way of helping. The commitment of the two young nursery nurses to the care of children became very evident and brought forth appreciative remarks from the teachers. The class teacher commented on the difficulty she sometimes had when concerned for a child whose parents were being helped by another worker whom she never saw. The senior social worker commented that she was glad the teacher had said this because, when social workers were up to their eyes in work, it was easy for them to overlook the contributions and concern of other workers. Finally it was agreed that the nursery staff would treat Mrs Anson like all the other mothers; that she should bring the children herself and if she were too late there would be no dinner for them. The nursery head would talk with her and explain the reasons for this rule.

A little while after the meeting, the nursery head said to the health visitor that she was glad she had brought her two young workers with her to the conference, although it had left the nursery short-staffed. She was also glad she had delayed the proceedings in order to discuss and clarify with them the social worker's aims. The nurses had felt that their views were taken into account and now had a much better understanding of the situation as a whole. She felt they were carrying out the agreed policy with a will and not just because they had been told to. She added: 'If they had not agreed with it, they would certainly have found ways of undermining it'.

This example shows a number of typical causes of collaborative failure. First, failure to enlist the user's active collaboration at the beginning. Although Mrs Anson went along with the plans for her children she was not encouraged to be an active participant in the planning. Inevitably she must have felt herself to be marginalised; and she was encouraged into, rather than helped out of, the role of the inadequate person. It was necessary for the professionals to take on some responsibility for the children in this case, but it was not necessary to undermine the mother's sense of responsibility.

Second, there was a failure to recognise the need for an integrated *help-compact*. I find it necessary to introduce this new term to describe the help as a whole which, at any one time, is being offered to the user. I prefer the word *compact* to that of 'package', which is sometimes used, because optimal help is never a packaged product. It is always individually prepared and involves all three aspects of the word 'compact', which is defined as: 'a covenant, a structure, a composition'; 'to compact' meaning 'to join or knit firmly together'. It may be either a *help-compact* or a *care-compact*. In my work help has predominated so I tend to use the former, but in other fields care-compact may be the more appropriate term.

If it had been recognised at the beginning that the tasks and responsibilities of those involved needed to be closely integrated, an initial meeting might have been called, including the headteacher, education welfare officer, social worker, health visitor and nursery head and, for at least part of the time, the mother. The latter would then have been an active participant. A common approach could have been worked out, responsibilities clarified, and the necessary lines of communication established.

An initial meeting to prepare a compact usually involves fewer people than a later meeting to sort out a muddle. Here, it would only have been necessary for the nursery head to attend because she could then have put over an agreed policy to her staff. When a meeting is called at a later stage, people who have become subsequently involved may need to be included in the discussions which precede a change of plan, otherwise they may not be convinced of the rightness of the decisions taken and be unwilling to carry them out. Sorting out a collaborative muddle at a later stage usually involves more working hours than would have been spent on effective collaboration at the beginning.

If the mother had been included in an initial meeting she would have had the opportunity to participate as a self-helper and a collaborator with an active role. Instead she was encouraged into an increasingly dependent and inferior role which she began to exploit. We see a piecemeal plan, each agency pursuing its own line of work, only partially integrated with that of the others, and the mother's central position and rightful role being quite unwittingly overridden by the helpers.

This was the situation until the social worker realised her mistake. However, she did not see the active involvement of the mother as a new development in an agreed help-compact, so it did not occur to her to communicate this to the other workers. Hence the third cause of failure in collaboration: lack of adequate communication. This resulted in the aims of one worker being unwittingly undermined by the aims of another. Only the health visitor, who had at one time been the sole worker, seemed alert to the need for an integrated compact.

A further common hindrance to collaboration, illustrated here, is failure to appreciate the contribution of other faceworkers. The identification that the class teacher felt with the nursery nurses for being out of touch with the worker helping the mother of children in their care, brought to light the shared feeling that their work was undervalued. It led to explicit acknowledgement of their contribution. This clarification of feeling followed on the owning of a fault by the social worker. Faceworkers are naturally afraid to admit a mistake, but – and this is an important proviso – where there is sufficient basic goodwill, leading to security and open communication in a well-chaired group, it always seems to increase mutual understanding. In a rather similar case, the social worker, after acknowledging that she had acted over-hastily, explained that it was the result of her great anxiety about children at risk. The other workers immediately responded sympathetically. Defensive covering up usually produces an unsympathetic response and blocks the sorting-out process which leads to increased fellow-feeling.

When a help-compact has been planned collaboratively, the actual provision of help is more likely to be successful. However, this does not always happen, as is shown in the next case.

Bill Bowles, a rehousing failure

> **A** psychiatrist had gone to great trouble to help an in-patient, Bill Bowles, obtain a flat from a local housing association. Collaboration between the workers at the initial stages had been good, but it was only when Bill was suddenly readmitted to hospital that it was seen to have been insufficient. When contact was made with the housing association, it was found that Bill had been infringing tenancy conditions to the annoyance of other tenants, and had continued to do so despite warnings. The problem had not been communicated to the psychiatric department, the housing worker trying to deal with the situation herself, according to her usual methods, until one night a crisis blew up and a neighbouring tenant called the police. Only after re-admission was contact re-established between the psychiatric department and the housing worker. The latter then said that the tenancy must be terminated, because she had to consider the effect on the other tenants if she were too lenient with Bill.

Here the immediate cause of failure was the absence in the original compact of a procedure for continuing communication between the hospital and housing association workers. Not only did the failure affect Bill's chance of independent living, it also soured relationships between the two agencies, and reduced the possibility of future collaborative ventures. Bad feeling was engendered because the housing workers felt that they had not been sufficiently warned of possible difficulties, and the psychiatrist felt that the problem need not have escalated if he had been informed at the time it first arose. Both complaints seem justified, and a further hindrance to collaboration is exposed: that of mutual recrimination without an adequate attempt to understand the other worker's point of view. Failure to sort out difficulties and misunderstandings prevents positive use being made of a bad situation in order to establish a better working relationship in the future.

> **W**hen the psychiatrist was telling the ward sister what had happened, she said that Bill was at the moment trying to see how far he could go in breaking ward rules. That morning he had laid in bed, daring the nurses to make him get up,

whilst the other patients looked on with keen interest. He made the nurses angry and they had felt like telling him to get up or get out.

Behind the inadequate collaboration there is a deeper cause to the rehousing failure. This was the 'repeating pattern' in which Bill was caught and which became apparent in the discussion between psychiatrist and ward sister. Once seen, it could be used to help Bill understand his self-defeating behaviour which had been a pattern through much of his life. Unfortunately it was too late to retain the tenancy.

Repeating patterns stem from early family relationships which become incorporated in personality structure. A user may project a parental figure on to a worker holding a position of authority. Workers may get drawn into the situation and the old pattern will then be re-enacted. Here the reactive anger of the nurses with Bill Bowles throws light on the strong negative reaction of the housing worker. Thus a subtle cause of collaborative failure stems from the user's unwitting input. Where a user's past has contained much parental dispute, there may be an unrecognised need to recreate this same pattern between the workers, who may unexpectedly find themselves at loggerheads.

The relational patterns of users may also have a very subtle influence on the relationships of workers, through a *mirroring process*. In this a current family situation is played out unwittingly by workers. The following example illustrates this and, in addition, the problem of identifying the user. When working with children it is always important to consider whether the family as a unit should be considered the user, including both parents and other children, rather than the child alone, with the parents in a subsidiary role.

Clare Cooke, the symptomatic schoolgirl

The following story was pieced together at a meeting called by an education welfare officer, at the request of the headteacher:

Clare was a girl of 11 in her first year at a comprehensive school. Her attendance was always poor and after a while she began on occasion to feel ill in class, when she would be sent to the sick-bay. Here the nurse let her lie down and if Clare felt she could not go back into class phoned her mother to collect her. The class teacher had brought up the subject of these absences with the house tutor. He found Clare difficult to get to know, but she told him she liked her class and had no particular problems in school. He wrote asking both parents to come to see him but only the mother came. Mrs Cooke was co-operative; she seemed to be in comfortable circumstances with no particular problems, but a nervous person. She said that her husband started early for work and she then got Clare off to school. The latter was becoming increasingly difficult about going. She had been very happy at her junior school and Mrs Cooke had known all the teachers there. It was arranged that the school doctor should see Clare, and the examination showed her to be quite healthy. The pattern continued, and from time to time Clare would not even turn up at school, occasional doctor's certificates being sent.

Eventually the problem was brought to the notice of the head of the lower school who asked both parents to see him, but only the mother came. The latter said that when Clare did not go to school, in order to get some fresh air and be doing something useful, she would go to a neighbour who bred dogs and exercise them for her. Clare was very fond of this woman, and would spend quite a lot of time at weekends with her. The neighbour encouraged this, but Mrs Cooke added that her husband did not much like the neighbour. The headmaster suggested to Mrs Cooke that she take a firmer line with Clare, and he discussed this with the education welfare officer. The result was that Clare came to school more regularly but still frequented the sick-bay and went home early.

At the meeting the GP said that he often prescribed tranquilisers for Mrs Cooke and because he knew her so well he would sometimes repeat these without seeing her. He did not think there was much wrong with Clare but had given sick notes occasionally, when she had had flu or a tummy upset. He was glad to discuss the matter and would now be alerted to the situation.

In a review some months later it was found that nothing had changed. The question arose as to whether Clare should be referred to a child guidance clinic. It was decided to discuss this possibility with the parents. The school knew that the clinic's policy was to see both parents, so the education welfare officer visited in the evening to explain this to the father. Only then did it become apparent that Mrs Cooke had not told her husband about their daughter's problem. He was angry and insisted on seeing the headmaster. From this point the situation began to change, and referral to the child guidance clinic was ultimately found unnecessary.

In this case there appeared to be good collaboration between mother, child and school staff and between the staff themselves. What was discovered to be lacking was the father's collaboration. When a problem arises it is important to identify the user, and this may take time. In many school situations the primary user is the child. Here, however, through the helping process, it became clear that the potential user – the one in need of help – was the family, and Clare's behaviour was a symptom of family dysfunction. Help was ineffective until collaboration of the user-unit – the family – was engaged.

In the education welfare officer's subsequent discussions with the two parents together it emerged that the father and mother were estranged, having little communication. The mother compensated for this by an over-close relationship with her daughter, encouraging the girl's detachment from her father. With hindsight it is possible to see the mirroring process in operation – the family pattern being reflected within the school. The sick-bay nurse did not confer with the house tutor, who happened to be a man, about how to help Clare get back into class, but instead she phoned the mother. When this was pointed out in a later discussion the nurse said she was surprised at herself, because it was not her usual way of going about things. She then realised that Clare's mother had been insistent that she should be phoned if Clare seemed unwell, and she herself had fallen in with this rather than following her usual pattern of first approaching a child's tutor. Just as with a repeating pattern, recognition of a mirroring process not only frees the faceworker from its dominance but also offers a valuable aid to understanding the problem.

A third type of complication arises when faceworkers get caught up in strained agency, departmental or professional relationships. The following case involving faceworkers from two departments in a children's hospital shows how intergroup tensions can compound interpractitioner problems.

Daisy Daubney, the paediatric patient

A two-year-old child, Daisy, had been referred by the GP to the department of child psychiatry which had recently been transferred into the local hospital.

Daisy seemed to be withdrawn and not thriving, although physically fit. She was brought by her foster-mother who had looked after her for the past year, and who seemed a kindly and competent person, though saying she felt low at the moment because of difficulties in her marriage. Daisy was an illegitimate child of an SRN who worked as a sister in a hospital some distance away. The foster-mother said Mrs Daubney would not come to the hospital, so the psychiatric social worker saw her at the foster-home. The mother was a woman of rigid personality and strong religious faith. She felt extremely guilty about having an illegitimate child, and desperate that no-one in her profession should know. She felt very responsible and had made good arrangements for her daughter's care, but only came to visit her once a month and felt no affection for her. She was very upset that Daisy was not getting on well and keen that she should have the best attention, even if it meant paying for it. She gave details of the child's difficult first year, when she could not find a satisfactory foster-mother, and now she was worried because the present one had hinted that she might have to give up fostering.

The social worker said that the psychiatrist had wondered about having Daisy in hospital in order to observe her more closely but was hesitant to disrupt the relationship with the foster-mother and had decided to see the child again as an out-patient. Mrs Daubney said she would do all she could to help but could not come to the hospital as she was well-known in her profession and had always kept this child a secret. She enquired who saw the notes, and the social worker said that these were kept in the psychiatric department and not seen by the nurses.

A short time after this, at a weekend, Daisy was admitted to the hospital because of a respiratory infection with which the foster-mother felt unable to cope. Daisy therefore came under a paediatrician. It was agreed that the social worker attached to the child psychiatrist would continue with the case. She told the paediatrician of the mother's situation and explained that she had contact with her, meeting her at the foster-home. While Daisy was in hospital it became evident that she was very backward and withdrawn, and the question of placement was under discussion. Meanwhile the infection was cured and the child was to be discharged. One of the junior doctors approached the social worker asking her to get the mother to come to the hospital so that the child could be discharged into her care. The social worker explained that there was a difficulty and said there seemed no reason why Daisy could not be discharged to the foster-mother, as the child had been admitted on her authority. Later the same morning the paediatric consultant sent for the social worker who by this time was seeing a client, and sent a message back that she would come as soon as she was free. When they met both were on edge. The social worker explained her reasons for not forcing Mrs Daubney to attend the hospital and said she would get any necessary forms signed. The paediatrician said that he always liked to see a parent at the time of discharge and he had never had any difficulty with the social worker attached to his unit in arranging this. Neither was prepared to give way. The situation was finally resolved by the case being transferred to the psychiatrist who then discharged the child into the foster-mother's care.

Both paediatrician and psychiatric social worker were upset, neither having been in such a position before, wondering why the situation had escalated and whether they could have done anything to prevent it. They both trusted the paediatric social worker and came to her separately with their side of the story, which tallied factually. The psychiatric social worker said that the paediatrician had expected her to come and see him immediately, but she had just started on an interview with a distressed mother and was not going to interrupt it, so she had kept him waiting for about three-quarters of an hour. The consultant psychiatrist would not have expected her to do otherwise. The paediatrician seemed to think social workers were at his beck and call. He did not have any thought for the feelings of the mother, and was only concerned with formal procedures.

The consultant said to the paediatric social worker that no social worker had ever kept him waiting for three-quarters of an hour; he had thought she would only be a few minutes, so he waited around and this made him late for his next clinic. She did not seem to realise how busy he was. He respected social workers and always listened to them, but she appeared so sure that she was right. Perhaps the child psychiatrist encouraged this sort of attitude, he certainly was very free and easy in the way he spoke with the nurses.

Piecing together the two views of the one episode it became clear that the problem had first arisen out of a mismatch of expectations between the practitioners based on their previous experience of the other's profession which had been limited to relationships in a particular setting: the paediatrician's to hospital social workers; the psychiatric social worker's to a child psychiatrist in a setting outside the hospital. Further trouble had been created by inadequate communication, the social worker's message not conveying how long she would be. The irritation caused by a worker from child psychiatry touched off latent irritation concerning the transfer of child psychiatry from its previously detached site into the hospital; departmental rivalries were active and the question of psychiatric beds on the paediatric ward was a sensitive subject currently under discussion between the consultants. These tensions, although not directly related, compounded the difficulties between the two practitioners.

> The paediatric social worker was distressed by such a gross failure in collaboration. She could identify with the social worker's point of view about Mrs Daubney but she had a great respect for the paediatrician and knew him to be sensitive to the feelings of parents. She knew that he was formal in his ways and that the child psychiatrist had a very different style. She understood why the psychiatric social worker had failed in a situation in which she herself would have had no problem.

If the two practitioners had previously worked together the difficulties of this case would have been offset by a personalised working relationship, containing feelings of mutual trust and respect. This being absent and departmental tensions being present, they both reacted in a defensive pattern. Feeling their position was misunderstood and undervalued by the other, each was impelled to uphold their professional status: the social worker stood by her opinion, the doctor by his authority. Here we see a number of common causes of collaborative failure. First, a mismatch of expectations, arising from ignorance in both workers about the behavioural norms of another agency; second, incomplete communication leading to a misapprehension and consequent muddle; third, current intergroup tensions compounding the difficulties. Together these factors presented a formidable barrier to collaborative work.

Professional status can also be the cause of difficulties in collaboration between members of the same profession particularly when they are attached to different agencies, as the following example shows.

Eddy Edwards. the day centre member

> A psychiatrist who held out-patient clinics at the local hospital referred many cases to the day centres and psychiatric hostel run by the social services

department. From time to time he held a meeting with their heads, and he was always ready to discuss a case if they contacted him.

Difficulties arose when the community psychiatric nursing team was being developed. The psychiatrist devolved some of his work to the nurses, particularly where they were administering drugs on a long-term basis. The centre heads made an effort to adjust to the new situation and to relate well to the CPNs whose work they appreciated. The head who found this most difficult was the one who had a nursing qualification. She had been used to working closely with doctors and she valued her relationship with the psychiatrist. She found it unsatisfactory that contact with him was now sometimes replaced by contact with a nurse. Although she knew that the Community Psychiatric Nurse was dealing with certain centre members, she would find reasons for bypassing her and phoning the psychiatrist. The CPN became increasingly restive and appealed to the psychiatrist not to take such calls but refer them to her. The psychiatrist felt loyalty to both workers, and tried not to take calls from the centre head when he could find a way of doing so without appearing to be avoiding her.

There came a time when Eddy Edwards, a regular attender at the centre, did not turn up for several days. The centre head, although she knew the CPN was involved, decided to send a centre worker to visit him at home. This worker spoke with both Eddy and his mother. The latter said her son had lately begun to feel unsettled at the centre and less keen to attend. Mrs Edwards added that he seemed more withdrawn and that she had been thinking of asking for an appointment with the psychiatrist. The worker wondered why Mrs Edwards had not approached the centre to discuss the change in her son. She replied that the CPN had said she should no longer have contact with the centre but talk to her instead. At this moment Eddy entered the room, recognised the centre worker and went out again. The worker said that perhaps she could talk to Eddy, and his mother fetched him back. In reply to the worker's opening remark, he said: 'I see you at the centre'. 'I know', she said, 'but today I've come to see you at home'. He replied: 'But the nurse does that'. Mrs Edwards said that this suddenly reminded her of when she and her husband had separated and Eddy always needed to know exactly which of them he saw where. 'I think he is upset by your coming here', she added and, turning to her son, told him he should be pleased the lady had taken the time to come and see him. He thanked the worker for coming and mumbled something that she thought included the words 'It's not right'. She herself felt that something was not right and that anything she said might make it worse. Soon she left.

This visit caused a row between the centre head and the CPN and brought the problem into the open. It was clear to each of them that the person they were both trying to help was suffering as a result of their bad relationship. Each felt it was the other's attitudes and actions that caused the trouble. When the CPN said that she did not have nearly as much difficulty with the other centre heads they became alerted to the nature of their problem, and agreed that they must try and find a way to resolve it.

In most cases of poor collaboration the user is likely to suffer, but this case shows how much a vulnerable user, without having any clear idea of the cause of his distress, may be disturbed by a bad relationship between face-workers.

Professional status, measured here by contact with the consultant, is one element in the problem. Underlying this is another factor – reaction to the development of a new professional specialism. New specialist workers are always concerned with defining their sphere of functioning, some of which is theirs alone, whilst other parts overlap the domain of existing faceworkers. Any professional or agency development always affects existing boundaries and however much the development may be welcomed in principle in practice it is almost inevitably experienced by some group of workers as an infringement of their domain. If the problems resulting from change cannot be fully worked out between those concerned, collaboration is bound to be difficult. Since bad feeling tends to find an outlet somewhere, if workers do not handle hostility when it arises between them other people are liable to get caught up in the negative process. The problem may get lodged in users who become pawns in a power game. When the two workers removed the problem from Eddy and confronted it together they manifested another familiar hindrance to collaboration: they both agreed that change was necessary and they both thought it was for the other to make the changes.

Differences between faceworkers may also arise from conflicting views on how to help. Where this has been recognised before a new worker is introduced the differences may be worked out in advance. If unrecognised, the help offered may not only be less effective but an additional problem may be created for the user, who becomes the recipient of other people's conflicting views.

The Foster family, smoking teenagers

A GP referred a family, the Fosters, to a child guidance clinic because the two elder boys were getting into trouble with the police. In the course of the first family interview the parents blamed the school for being too easy on the boys, but it soon became apparent that the father had little control himself and the discussion revolved round the problem of authority in the family. The psychiatrist helped them to discuss what control was needed and how it should be enforced; in making practical suggestions the children themselves seemed keen for their father to assert himself more, and the psychiatrist encouraged this.

In the second family interview, Mr Foster reported on methods he had tried for enforcing his authority. Mrs Foster appeared to have upheld her husband, saying that she agreed he should stop the boys' pocket money if they continued to disobey him and also if they did not help in the home in the way she thought they should. However, as the family continued to talk, the youngest boy interjected: 'But, Mum, you did give Terry money for fags'. A shocked pause followed this disclosure. Mrs Foster then explained that recently when she had been to see her GP about her headaches the latter had asked about the boys and she had sought his advice on their smoking. He had suggested a policy of leniency as the most likely way of preventing them from making it a habit. Mrs Foster trusted her GP and had never gone against his advice. She had discussed this with her husband who wanted to continue on the line suggested by the psychiatrist, but agreed to turn a blind eye to the smoking. The ensuing discussion uncovered a subtle subversion by the mother of the father's authority within the family. This was a pattern of long-standing which had been disturbed by the intervention of the child psychiatrist. With unwitting backing from her GP Mrs Foster could have prolonged the old pattern if it had not come to light.

This shows how differences between practitioners can be unintentionally exploited by users to support their maladaptive behaviour. It was possible because of insufficient collaboration between workers providing concurrent help. The two faceworkers had not considered the need for working out an integrated help-compact until the little boy uncovered the lack of collaboration between them. Only then did the doctors begin to clarify their different tasks within the overall task of helping the family.

When the problem of divergent views between workers becomes lodged in the family, workers will be unaware of the family's conflict until it is presented to one or other of them. This kind of situation is particularly likely to occur where users have a dependent and passive attitude when seeking help, and where workers have unwittingly encouraged it through taking a particularly active or dominant role.

Deliberate lack of communication leading to negative consensus is at the root of failure in collaboration in the following example.

Mrs Gould, the paranoid mother

A case conference was held about a family, the Goulds, who had been referred to a department of child psychiatry by the education welfare department, because of the disturbed state of the two little girls and the fact that the younger one was learning very little. At the conference the psychiatrist said she had found Mrs Gould very critical of the school, blaming the headmaster and class teacher for the younger child's lack of progress. Mrs Gould was found to be paranoid and greatly in need of help herself, but very resistant to any such suggestion and loath to bring her children to the hospital again. The psychiatrist thought the children should be taken into care, but legal opinion in the social services department advised against attempting such action. Finally as an interim plan it was agreed that the hospital social worker, who seemed to have made a good contact with Mrs Gould, should visit her at home and the school psychologist should see the children in school. A young education welfare officer had been visiting Mrs Gould and he agreed to call and explain that the hospital social worker would be taking his place and, after a further visit, would ease himself out.

At a second conference six months later it was found that he was still visiting regularly, unbeknown to the hospital social worker. He said: 'As I was frequently in that neighbourhood, I just dropped in from time to time'. When questioned about the purpose of his visit, he replied: 'I was concerned for the girls and I felt their mother needed more support than she was getting from the hospital'. On further discussion he disclosed that he had found Mrs Gould suspicious of the hospital social worker. The education welfare officer thought he had a better relationship with Mrs Gould and had more to offer her, but then he became worried when she began to think that he found her attractive. In the continuing discussion it became evident that he had thought Mrs Gould over-critical of the school but that he had fallen in with her mistrust of the hospital social worker. He began to express doubts about psychiatry in general, the methods of the department of child psychiatry and the social worker in particular. It then emerged that he had not been in agreement at the time the plan was formulated but had felt unable to voice his views.

 Here one worker lacked trust in another, and this was not brought out and discussed openly at the appropriate time. We do not know the basis for the education welfare officer's doubts. They may have had some validity; they may have come from his own past experiences or his general attitudes to psychiatric help, or from those of other people. He may also unwittingly have taken in some of Mrs Gould's feelings, thus increasing his own negative attitudes. These were not substantiated by the opinions of other workers present. It is not unusual for faceworkers to mistrust either the methods or the competence of other workers who are not personally well known to them. In addition, if there has been contact between a user and a faceworker over a period of time, it is not unusual for the latter to feel that another worker will not understand the user as well as they have done. Given these common phenomena it is essential that the compact is agreed as a result of positive consensus. Negative consensus – lip-service agreement covering unvoiced disagreement – cannot bring about effective collaboration.

These seven examples illustrate common collaborative difficulties. They are drawn from my particular experience, but the relational problems they describe will be familiar to faceworkers from all fields of help. Taken together they demonstrate the complexity of helping relationships and the subtle nature of hindrances to collaboration.

Chapter 3
A Relational Approach to Collaboration

The need

Although not disastrous the kind of collaborative failures described in the previous chapter have considerable negative repercussions. For users they lessen the effectiveness of help and sometimes add to distress; for face-workers they cause disappointment and frustration at the knowledge that users are badly served and time badly spent; for the helping services they lower standards and waste money. The question of how to eliminate or reduce their impact is increasingly urgent because the number of situations requiring facework collaboration is growing. This is the result of several causes.

First, an increase in services and options of help has resulted from the development of new specialisms and skills and the establishment of new projects or reshaping of old ones. When functions and services have been differentiated in order to provide effective and comprehensive help, it inevitably follows that, if more than one method of help is needed at any one time, there must be co-ordination. It may be possible to achieve this within the competence of one worker or within the functions of one setting but often this is impossible, owing to the great range of skills and services necessary for meeting many complex situations.

Second, there are a growing number of families which are either disorganised within themselves or not well integrated into the community and which have many-faceted troubles needing a wide range of help. Such families are found everywhere, but particularly in inner-city areas. Where needs are simple or where the individual or family is able to act as co-ordinator of the help if needed, routine collaboration between workers may be all that is necessary. However, in many cases the family is unable to organise the fulfilment of its own needs, thus increasing the need for facework collaboration. If unemployment is widespread complex problems become more prevalent.

Third, new social policies and changing attitudes are giving greater importance to the private sector, the community and the self-help movement. As a result of the growing emphasis on user participation and users' rights, along with other changes in society, people's expectations of

24

agencies and their attitudes to practitioners are changing. The professionals themselves are also changing in their attitudes to each other and to the community in which they work. The result is that long established patterns of helping relationships are now put in question.

To overcome the difficulties of collaboration, suggestions are sometimes made for restructuring professions; for instance, in mental health, the training of a 'mental health worker' who would combine both nursing and social work functions. This might eliminate some of the need for collaboration within the mental health field but, at the same time, it would increase the need for collaboration on other fronts – for instance, that between mental health and child care, since children are often at risk in families where there are mental health problems.

Hindrances to collaboration

Hindrances to collaboration can be reduced by efficient procedures and the development of organisational structures designed to facilitate transboundary relationships, such as health centres, the siting of various agencies in close proximity and multidisciplinary projects. However, restructuring professions and agencies can never provide the whole answer, and where there are complex problems there will always be a need for highly skilled collaboration between faceworkers. It is therefore essential to come to grips with the collaborative difficulties that stem from human relationships in the context of helping. To make a start, I classify the common causes of collaborative failure which arise from relational rather than organisational factors. Some of these have been illustrated in the previous chapter, others will be enlarged upon in later chapters.

Failure to identify the user
It is not always easy at the beginning of a helping situation to know whether the user-unit is an individual or a family, as was evident with the schoolgirl, Clare Cooke. However, because adults usually, and children always, are a member of a partnership or group, a natural or substitute family, faceworkers need to be alert to the possibility of the user being more than one person.

Failure to identify relevant people
Although not included in the user-unit, members of the extended family may well have a part in the situation, as may friends, neighbours or workmates with whom a user has a personal relationship. They may be contributing – negatively or positively – to the situation, and recognition of such relevant people is often important. The neighbour with the dogs was such a person in Clare's situation.

*Undervaluing the user as self-helper and diminishing their sense
of responsibility*
This is a common collaborative failure, the unfortunate results of which are
clearly illustrated in the case of Mrs Anson, the day nursery mother. If
responsibility is taken away from users unnecessarily, their contribution to
the help-compact is reduced and their status diminished.

Overlooking the user's unwitting input to the helping process
Repeating patterns and mirroring have been shown to influence the helping
process in the cases of Bill Bowles and his housing problem and the Cooke
family. Unrecognised, they cause problems in the collaborative relationships
either between user and faceworker, or between the faceworkers themselves, or both. Recognised, they are an invaluable aid to understanding the
situation and bringing about necessary change. Defensive processes in users
who attempt to get rid themselves of guilty feelings by blaming workers or
organisations, can disturb collaboration between faceworkers only if they
accept the user's view of the situation, without checking first, as happened in
the case of Mrs Gould, the paranoid mother.

Unawareness of the need for an integrated help-compact
In the case of Mrs Anson the need for collaboration did not appear to be part
of the thinking underlying the social worker's practice. She was the only
faceworker having links with all the other workers involved; and, since her
agency had a particularly important function in relation to the children,
responsibility seemed to fall on her to initiate the process for establishing an
integrated help-compact. It may be that the problem did not lie entirely in the
practitioner; the pressure and priorities of her agency may have made it
difficult for her to find time to organise a meeting, or even to discuss the
situation sufficiently fully with each worker on the phone.

An insufficiently integrated help-compact is also apparent in the case of
the Foster family and their teenage smokers. The GP did not see the need to
relate his input to that of the clinic to which he had referred the family. The
clinic workers did not think of the continuing input from the GP, and hence
the need for his approach to be integrated with that of the centre.

Failure to maintain a help-compact once established is seen in the case of
Bill Bowles. The housing worker did not feed back information to the
psychiatrist at the right time, to make it possible for him to intervene in a way
which might have contained a difficult situation. Complications often arise in
the course of helping, and maintaining an integrated help-compact is often
totally dependent on continuing collaboration.

Ignorance concerning other agencies and professions
Ignorance of the nature of another faceworker's task is illustrated in the case
of Bill Bowles. The psychiatrist did not appreciate the housing worker's need
to consider the tenants as a group as well as individually, although he

recognised a similar need within his hospital ward. Ignorance of behavioural norms is seen in the case of Daisy, the paediatric patient, the social worker being unfamiliar with hospital life; and in both faceworkers we see a mismatch of expectations, arising out of a narrow experience of the other's profession.

Often there is ignorance of the exact functions of other agencies, leading to inappropriate referrals. Often there is ignorance of their very existence. Failure to use an agency when its help could be useful is a common collaborative failing.

Narrow vision

Often help is not offered because the viewpoint of the initial helper is too narrow to take in the user's situation as a whole, and too restricted to a single profession or agency to encompass an overview of the help available. Such narrow vision may come from ignorance, lack of ability, defensiveness or a helping approach inadequate to the situation. It limits the help offered and prevents referrals.

Terminology

Professional terminology is necessary but it is important that practitioners ensure that the terms they use are properly understood by others. Where matters under discussion are part of the competence of several or all of the helping professions discussion is facilitated by a common terminology, but at present this is inadequate to collaborative needs and, in addition, confusion may arise from the same word being used in different ways. This hinders the process of mutual understanding, in that the assumptions made by practitioners from one discipline are not always apparent to practitioners from another.

Failures in communication

Failure to see the need for communication is an inevitable corollary of an inadequately integrated help-compact, as already noted in the cases of Mrs Anson, and the Foster family. Failure to establish adequate lines of communication for continuing collaboration, particularly where feedback is important, is frequently the cause of a well-established help-compact foundering later. This is illustrated in the outcome of Mr Bowles' rehousing. Confused communication leads to unnecessary muddles which disrupt collaboration. This was one factor in the breakdown of the working relationship between paediatrician and social worker in the case of Daisy.

Failure to convey relevant feelings and opinions means that communication is insufficiently open to reach a positive consensus. With negative consensus it is probable that certain decisions will not be implemented. In the case of Mrs Gould, if the education welfare officer's reservations had been brought into the open, some working through of hostile and suspicious feeling between faceworkers might have been possible. Then the decisions taken at the conference would have been implemented instead of undermined.

Lack of trust between faceworkers

Where faceworkers do not know each other it is inevitable that their initial reactions are to a stereotype; only gradually do the qualities of the particular faceworker become known and the relationship individualised. Thus it is natural for faceworkers to be cautious in the initial trust they accord. The image which a person attaches to a practitioner may be based on a generally held view, it may be personal or else borrowed from another worker or a user. If it is a negative one, it will be impossible to build up trust, as with the education welfare officer in the case of Mrs Gould. Only if mistrust can be dissipated will it be possible for collaborative relationships to develop. Frequently referrals are left unmade because of lack of trust in other workers or agencies. In the case of Daisy, mistrust was out in the open, leading to a total breakdown of collaboration. It cannot be overlooked that in such a case overt mistrust may turn out to be less harmful to the user than covert mistrust.

Rivalry between faceworkers

This can sometimes aid good practice through the effort to do a better job than someone else. However, when it is rivalry for position in a particular help-compact it can do nothing but harm. It reduces the possibility of collaboration and the conflict between workers is often experienced painfully by the user, as we saw with Eddy, the day centre member. Wherever the boundaries of tasks or skills are ill-defined the ground is ripe for the development of rivalry.

Conflicting opinions and attitudes

It is to be expected that practitioners will sometimes have differing opinions about what is likely to be helpful. These may not become apparent until a user brings them into the open, as in the case of the Foster family. At other times there may be open conflict. The attempt to resolve differences or to find a compromise is only likely to succeed if motivation to do so is strong and time is made for discussion.

It cannot be assumed that there is unanimity on the basic aims of helping nor, even where these are in accord, on their interpretation. In many cases such differences do not affect the help that is needed nor the collaborative process. Only when conflicting assumptions affect attitudes to the user or the choice of methods of help do fundamental differences of approach form a serious hindrance to collaboration.

Failure to own a fault and unresolved failures

In the case of Daisy and Bill Bowles, in order to keep themselves in the clear, each worker found it necessary to see the whole fault in the other, rather than owning some fault in themselves. This almost inevitably leads to mutual recrimination and deteriorating relationships.

If the cause of a failure is not sorted out it often leaves a bad taste that can sour relationships between the particular workers, and perhaps also between the agencies, for a long time to come – the *hangover effect*. If a collaborative failure can be worked through, with faults being owned, it can often lead to increased mutual understanding and improved working relationships. This process is seen in the meeting about Mrs Anson. It demands considerable integrity on the part of faceworkers and a situation in which there is basic goodwill.

Role-insecurity

Uncertainty in the working-role was experienced by the two faceworkers involved with Daisy. They were adjusting to organisational change, were the bearers of group rivalries concerning departmental boundaries, and involved in a working relationship which was unfamiliar to them. Role-insecurity is also caused by the distressing or intractable nature of the troubles presented; and the inability to help adequately, whether from lack of skill, lack of resources or because as yet there is no complete answer. This was evident in the discussion in the opening scene. A particular personal, as distinct from professional, anxiety may also cause a faceworker to feel insecure in certain situations. Role-insecurity, from whatever cause, is likely to lead to defensive reactions which hinder collaboration.

Defensive processes in faceworkers

These are often the response to situations which cause role-insecurity. Retreat behind professional and agency boundaries and their use as defences create major hindrances to collaboration. In the meeting about Mrs Anson, the social worker began to use a defensive pattern to justify her previous action, but was able to abandon it when challenged by the health visitor. The mutual recriminations of the psychiatrist and the housing worker in the case of Bill Bowles showed the common defensive process of keeping oneself in the clear by dumping inadequacy on the other side of the agency boundary. Defensive processes will be considered at length in Chapter 11.

Reaction to change

Changes almost inevitably cause insecurity. Organisational and professional restructuring were a factor in the case of Daisy, and Eddy. Currently some professions are being faced with formidable changes which include their relationships, on the one hand, to managers who are not trained in their own profession and, on the other, to less trained workers carrying out tasks which had been considered the sole province of their professional practice. Regardless of the rights and wrongs of any situation, change is likely to be accompanied by stress, resistance and defensive processes which hinder collaboration.

The viewing-point

This is the position from which helpers look at a situation. It is determined by their personal and/or professional values, attitudes and training; it can have a wide or narrow 'lens' in that it can take in a wide view or focus on a detail. This affects the kind of help that is offered, since it provides a standpoint from which situations are assessed, action taken and outcome evaluated. The following example shows the result of a widened viewing-point and more user-centred focus. It also shows how trust between workers can do much to neutralise mistakes and prevent their consequences escalating.

Mrs Hill, the depressed single parent

A GP had been treating a single parent, Mrs Hill, with antidepressants for some time when he decided to give her a longer session and encourage her to talk more about herself. She told him about her lonely life with one small child, isolated in a highrise block of flats. They agreed that he would ask a social worker to visit. The GP was beginning to enlarge his viewing-point and saw this as a social problem. He might have suggested contacting the health visitor who would have already been involved because of the young child. On the phone, the social worker suggested this and the GP said he was short of time. She got the impression that he would not make the contact, so agreed to accept the case and herself confer with the health visitor. The latter said that she had arranged for Mrs Hill to join a mother-and-toddlers' group but did not yet know how this had worked out; she was glad for the social worker to be involved as she felt the mother was depressed and needed more skilled counselling than she herself could offer. The two workers knew each other well, and they agreed that the GP's referral provided a reason for the social worker to visit.

Such an introduction of a new worker, particularly where skills overlap, can easily lead to confusion, rivalry and bad feeling. In this case, the health visitor knew that she was not as competent to help the mother as was the social worker; in another situation it could have been that the health visitor was the more skilled in counselling, and tasks would have been differently allocated. The personalised working relationship between the two practitioners was of value; without it, collaboration would have been a chancy affair. As it was, their mutual trust and respect made it easy to agree a help-compact.

The social worker visited and explained that she had been contacted by the GP and had spoken with the health visitor. Mrs Hill said she had felt out of it at the mother-and-toddlers' group, because she found herself unable to talk with the other mothers, and this made her feel even more lonely and depressed.

The social worker, after a few visits in which she helped Mrs Hill with her difficulties in getting to know people, suggested a self-help group for single parents. Here Mrs Hill was able to find companionship, partly because of her increased self-confidence, partly because the group was better suited to her situation. After a little while the social worker withdrew from the case, but before doing so arranged a brief meeting with the health visitor and GP, so that they made a link which could serve the future needs of the family. They continued this contact, and the GP's function of prescribing was integrated with the health visitor's work with mother and child. The help-compact was no longer fragmented and the medication was gradually reduced.

Many GPs have already developed an approach to primary health care which involves working closely with other helpers and making use of other agencies.Where this is not so, greater effort is required of other practitioners in initiating and maintaining a collaborative process.

Value-systems

In looking at the help offered to Mrs Hill certain values have been implicit. It is almost impossible to discuss helping without making value judgements. It can be assumed that within the personal helping services the general aim is the wellbeing of users, but people differ in their interpretation of this aim which influences their helping approach. The values of society, powerful organisations and pressure groups determine the services provided; and at the point of delivery, professional and personal values determine the actual help a user receives.

These value-systems are based on beliefs about human beings and society. Mine are that the human being is a unique physical, emotional, mental and spiritual organism with individual meaning and a social function. Helping is then evaluated on the basis of concern for the user's personal development within a social context. Wellbeing can then be more specifically formulated as: maximum self-responsibility, optimum quality of life, integration both personal and social. In future I refer to these criteria for measuring wellbeing as the *triple aim of helping*.

Self-responsibility implies that every user should, as far as possible and in a way that is compatible with the help that is needed, be looking after themselves and making their own decisions. If incapable for any reason, those nearest to them take charge wholly or in part, aided or substituted by helping organisations. Those who are dependent on others for care often have the capacity to exercise independence in certain areas of their life. Thus the allocation of tasks and responsibilities is always important. Capabilities change – damaged people improve or deteriorate, children and old people grow older – and the possibility of self-responsibility increases or diminishes. A sensitive reaction to changing circumstances is necessary in order to maintain the right balance of shared responsibility between user and helper.

In general terms, *quality of life* depends on a good self-image, some basic source of security, meaningful relationships and the opportunity to develop potential. It is for users to decide what enhances their quality of life, and it is for faceworkers to help a user to find and achieve this, subject to three provisos: it must be within the law, within limits set by the overall help available and the needs of other users and by the needs of personal carers. Concurrently with that of the user, the wellbeing of personal carers and other members of the family must be taken into account. Subject to these limitations, users are entitled to help from below par up to their own previous level or to that of the average citizen or family – what might be termed *personal par* and *average par*.

Where users are not in a position to interpret the meaning of 'quality of life' for themselves, this task will fall to others. Although it may be comparatively easy to formulate general criteria for wellbeing, the interpretation in any particular situation, especially if made on behalf of someone else, may be far from easy. In reaching a balanced view, collaboration between personal carers and practitioners is particularly important.

Personal integration means helping a user achieve a sufficiently harmonious internal state to be able to have meaningful relationships and function adequately. *Social integration* contributes to this objective, so that there is value in help that relates an individual or family to their local community rather than isolating them from it. This means that where they wish to join in local life they are welcomed and encouraged, and where their preferred way of life is that of a recluse they are accepted.

These three aims of helping are interwoven: for example, self-responsibility can be better exercised by a well integrated person. Shared responsibilities between a user and a carer can give added meaning to their relationship; when looking back over troubles faced together, couples sometime say that their lives have been enriched in quite unforeseen ways. Quality of life is often enhanced through social integration, resulting in a sense of belonging within a group or community.

The integrative approach to helping

A helping approach is based on values, ideology and attitudes concerning helping. They may be very different, or they may overlap with each other. I propose one which I call the *integrative approach*. Its core is the user-centred model, the triple aim of helping and the integrated help-compact. Based on a holistic approach, it incorporates a family approach, in which the individual is viewed as part of a family or other group, and the family as belonging to a cultural background and functioning in a social setting. It interprets a community approach as meaning not only caring for people in their own home or within their local community, but also maintaining the user's self-responsibility and social integration, giving weight to the needs of the carer and family as well as those of the user, and developing networks of local help.

The relational component in this overall helping approach is essential and extensive. It leads to the interpretation of collaborative care as including not only practitioners, paid workers, personal carers, but also volunteers, self-help groups, local people, family and friends; and, with few exceptions, the user as self-helper and participant in the helping process.

Chapter 4
Provision of Help and Helping Relationships: Collaborative Framework I

I have found that discussion between different disciplines and agencies is often bedevilled by the lack of a common base from which to start, so here, as well as amplifying the meaning of an integrative approach, I describe certain concepts and define the way in which I use some familiar terms that have subtle variations of meaning.

Sources of help

Help and *care* are often used as interchangeable words but although their meanings overlap they are not synonymous. Both are the realm of the helping services. As I use the term, care means looking after, with human concern, through tending and protecting. It implies a position of ability and responsibility in the carer, in relation to some lack of capacity in the user. Help implies a more specific input in assisting users to improve or at least maintain their situation. It does not imply such an imbalance of capacity, as does 'care'. In the present context each includes aspects of the other: care includes helping, and helping includes caring. Sometimes one, sometimes the other predominates and seems the more appropriate term.

Fields of help are the seven broad areas of help which cover: the dependency of children and the elderly, physical health, mental health, disability, social disadvantage and social maladjustment.

The provision of help is dependent on resources. These are: institutional – organisational structures and buildings; material – financial and physical aids, drugs, etc.; human – people with the capacity to organise or provide help.

Formal care is provided by the statutory and fully organised voluntary (sometimes called independent) agencies and the private sector. The *statutory services* include the local authority's social services department and services run by national authorities – the NHS and Department of Social Security. The *voluntary organisations* are set up by concerned people to meet a particular need. The formal ones are well structured, run by an executive committee, funded by voluntary contributions or charities but probably also by grants from statutory bodies, and registered as a charity. An

34

example of those organised on a national basis is the NSPCC; on a local basis, but affiliated to a national body, are the local associations of MIND. Functioning solely on a local basis, there are many smaller organisations, well-organised and having charitable status. The *private sector* may be run on a profit making or non-profit making basis. The formal services have grown up over the centuries through the development of specialised methods and professions. Gradually they have fallen into two main systems – *health care* and *social care*, which I distinguish as physical and psychological on the one hand, social and psychological on the other.

Formal care is provided through *agencies*. Many organisations function through a single agency, others have a number of agencies acting as outlets for their services. Viewed from the top, these outlets might be seen as sub-agencies of a single agency. Viewed from ground level, provided they are making their own relationships locally, they are likely to be seen as agencies in their own right, coming under a supra-agency. The degree of autonomy of such agencies may be of considerable importance to their own and other workers when collaborating at ground level. The structures of agencies are varied but can be classified within three main types of help-setting: *in-care*, which includes hospitals and residential homes; *day care*, which includes day centres, day hospitals and drop-in centres; and *out-care*. This may be provided in an *out-centre*, such as hospital out-patients, GP surgery, social work office, drop-in centre; through *home care*; or through *out-reach care*, when workers search out those who need help wherever they may be.

I have spelt out what most readers already know because I wish to draw attention to the influence the set-up of the services has on the relationships of their workers. Every agency is a system with a boundary across which negotiations have to take place when collaboration with other agencies is needed. It can never be assumed that two agencies, although working in the same field, have identical objectives. This was made clear to me when hospital social workers were transferred from the health service to their local social services department. They became accountable to, and staff were appointed by, a different organisation and its management. Instead of being members of the hospital staff they became a sub-agency of the social services department with its own priorities. Relationships between the medical and social work practitioners gradually changed; certain assumptions about the social worker's role could no longer be made and were replaced by specific negotiation. This highlighted the complex connections between the two important boundaries of agency and profession and the way in which they affect the identification and relationships of the practitioner.

Informal care refers to the help provided by individual people – family and friends; and by the local community – neighbours or helpers in small informal voluntary agencies or groups. These have minimal structure and budgets – for example, a group formed to take people with handicaps to the swimming-baths.

Formal and informal care also includes that provided within organisations set up for ordinary life purposes, such as schools, churches, information services, community or recreational groups. Besides the specific structures which some of them provide as part of the formal helping services – such as the school medical service, various counselling services or housing for special needs – some of their workers or members, in the course of pursuing their ordinary aims, help with troubles which also come the way of the helping services. This may happen incidentally or intentionally. For example, a social worker having contact with an adult education institute may enlist the assistance of their teachers in giving special help to a user wishing to get back into formal education. Because the organisations of everyday life supplement the helping services, I class them as *para-helping organisations*.

The community

It is essential to be clear what is meant by the word since it is used in many different ways.

Whose community?

In a group including workers from inside and outside a hospital, a discussion grew increasingly heated and confused, until it became evident that people were talking at cross-purposes. When using the phrase 'in the community' hospital workers were referring to all services and workers outside the hospital; whilst the latter were meaning people and groups in the local neighbourhood. It was a social worker whose identifications spanned the hospital boundary who clarified this. A hospital doctor then said: 'But I think of the hospital as a community. It feels like that to me. We have a community of interest and are a very united group of people'. A hospital social worker replied: 'But I think of the hospital as being in the community – it is a district hospital and it belongs to the neighbourhood'.

All these ways of using the word 'community' are valid. There can be a number of different communities covering or within the same locality, some embracing others, some mutually exclusive. Communities may be territorially based, such as the county, borough and neighbourhood; others are institutionally-based, such as a hospital, day or residential centre; yet others are based on social bonds, such as a common culture, race or religion. For a working definition of the term *community* I propose: a group of people who feel at one with each other on the basis of a common existential bond, either territorial (living or working in the same area) institutional (living or working together in a common establishment or organisation, whether or not housed in one building) characteristic (sharing personal or social characteristics of a strong, durable and recognisable nature) or of a strongly shared interest. Whenever the word is used it is essential that everyone understands to which particular community they are referring.

Territorial communities can be large or small, ranging from the EU to a single street and the local community. Here I am only concerned with the latter – an area to which residents or workers can in some way feel a sense of belonging. Within it, local community organisations and groups may be formed by people with other common bonds. By way of illustration, in the area covered by the London Borough of Kensington and Chelsea, people seem to feel they belong not so much to the borough as a whole as to, say, Notting Hill, South Kensington, Earls Court, Chelsea, the World's End Estate, etc. Within an estate, there may be still smaller communities, relating to a street or staircase of a block of flats. Covering these local communities or within them there may be others based on common characteristics or on institutions; in Notting Hill, for instance, the black community, Moroccan community, the community of churches, a residential therapeutic community.

Local communities can be given assistance for their development and rehabilitation. Although I do not discuss this, I wish to stress its importance and bearing on the personal helping services. Some individual and family troubles would never arise if communities were functioning well. It is obvious that when good water supplies and sewerage are provided certain kinds of personal ill-health disappear. Community wellbeing covers much more than public health and has far-reaching effects on the wellbeing of individuals and families, their physical and mental health, personal and social quality of life. Community wellbeing has a bearing on the ways in which the troubles of its members can be helped, and can be a valuable source of personal help.

The helpers

The terms helper, worker and carer, often refer to the same person, but sometimes one seems more appropriate, sometimes another. If workers are defined as people who do something useful, whether or not they are employed or paid, then all helpers are workers. They are either formal or informal carers according to where they work. *Informal carers* include: *personal carers* – family, friend or neighbour – who help as the result of a personal bond; and *local carers*, volunteers in informal community groups. However, although the care many informal carers provide is similar to that of the helping services, they do not wish to be considered as part of them because their caring stems from their personal relationship. They have come to be known as '*the carers*'. Although service workers are carers and personal carers are workers, for the sake of clarity, I use the term 'carer' to refer to the personal carers, and 'worker' to refer to those employed in helping agencies or working privately.

Workers include practitioners of all the helping professions, trained and untrained workers, care-workers, and those volunteers working in helping organisations. The boundary between trained workers and practitioners is not clearly defined, particularly in fields where methods and skills are developing.

All helpers except the self-helper are included in the term faceworker. The *self-helper* is a distinct category of helper in that they are also the user; here the interface between user and helper is an internal one. When self-helpers with similar problems get together they may be the helper or the one helped, or both simultaneously; in fact they become *mutual helpers*. Formed into a *self-help group*, the interface between user and helper is internal to the group.

Methods of help

A method of help or *help-method* is a defined process using institutional, material and/or human resources, developed to meet particular kinds of situation. Often differentiated as medical or social, they can also be classified according to other factors; for example, *practical* or *relational methods*, if one or the other aspect predominates. Focusing on the location of the main helping input, other classifications would be into: *setting methods*, in which the place – such as a residential unit – and the user's relation to it and to the other residents has an important function; *facework methods*, in which the faceworker's skills are crucial; and *practice methods*, when the competence of a practitioner is essential.

The three main types of help are care, treatment and enablement. Care means looking after, with human concern, through tending and protecting. It relies heavily on the setting methods of in-care, daycare and homecare, and on facework methods. Where protection is required practice methods are always needed. *Treatment* means specific skilled intervention. It includes many medical methods, but some social methods fall into this category, such as intermediate treatment and behaviour therapy. *Enablement* is the overall term I use to describe non-specific intervention which actively engages users in finding solutions to their own troubles and helps them to help themselves. Enablement includes a number of well-tried methods. In problem-solving, help draws on the user's own resources, which may be supplemented by service resources. Through rights entitlement, help is given to ensure that users are in receipt of the assistance to which they are entitled. Personal and family support is designed to help users cope and keep going, backing up their strengths through encouragement and/or other types of help. Group participation helps a user to develop a greater ability to relate and cope, through building relationships and sharing activities. Counselling helps users develop a well-adapted response to a particular situation through clarifying the issues involved, enabling them to express their feelings, understand their emotional reactions and the personal inter-actions which are relevant to their situation. There are many types of rela-tional psychotherapy which are all enablement methods aiming to assist personal and social integration. Methods of treatment have been mainly developed within health care for physical troubles, and methods of enable-ment within social care for socially orientated troubles. However, as both spheres are concerned with psychological care there is a large area of overlap. Here because of the lack of definition, there is confusion and wide scope for rivalry.

Methods always have objectives which, for all three categories of help, can be defined and measured according to the *user's capability-level*. This can be graded as: return to normal, either average or personal par; improved; maintained; adjusted to a lower level; or dignified deterioration. Capability-level applies to physical, emotional, mental and social functioning. When it comes to a choice of method, objectives based on level of capability in these four areas may have to be weighed according to the values held by user and/or faceworker. For example, drug treatment for a psychological trouble may help a person to function better but psychotherapy, counselling, behaviour therapy, group participation or other methods of enablement might be the treatment of choice, on the grounds that as well as bringing about better functioning over time they offer a better quality of life for the user.

Help-compact and helping-task

I have used *trouble* as a comprehensive term to cover physical, emotional, mental, personal and social – needs, problems, difficulties, disorders, dis-ability, disadvantage and maladjustment. The *presenting trouble* is the one for which the user seeks help. There may be an *underlying trouble* which is causally connected with it and which could receive attention, should the faceworker identify it and the user wish to focus on it. In addition there may be *concurrent troubles*, which were not presented initially but which might be found to need help. Finally there is the *target trouble*, the one which is actually made the focus of help. If help is to be adequate, users and their troubles may need to be seen in the context of their life *situation*. This is composed of the user, the trouble, the current relationships and general position in which the user is placed.

The *help-compact* that is provided to meet the needs of the situation may be a single method of help or several methods integrated into a whole. It may be brief, short-term or long-term, the latter being continuous or periodic, that is, requiring help at intervals only. The help-compact has various stages. Initial and early stages include assessment, planning and decision-making; middle stages cover implementation of the plan; final stages include review and ending, with or without follow-up and option to return. There may be interim reviews, reassessment, referral and transition from one setting, method or faceworker to another. The progression is simple in a mono-phase compact, which is either a brief intervention or, if longer, a situation in which everything remains unchanged. In a multiphase compact, methods change along with changing situations in the helping process.

Whereas the help-compact covers all kinds of resources and defines the methods employed, the *helping-task* refers solely to human resources – the input of user and faceworkers. It is the sum of human activity necessary for carrying out a particular help-compact. For every helping-task there is a level of *minimum essential collaboration*, or *MEC*. This means the mini-mum number of people with the necessary competence for the task, using the minimum amount of their time to achieve it. Many methods of help require the integration of human resources with institutional or material resources. Other methods, such as counselling or advice-giving, only require human input; then the helping method and the helping-task are identical.

Within the helping-task as a whole – the *overall task* – there will be a number of *constituent* or what I define as *work-tasks* to specify the parti-cular task a particular person is carrying out. Just as methods need to be integrated to make an effective help-compact, so constituent tasks need to be 'confected' to make the helping-task effective. I have found the need to introduce this term to describe the subtle process of combining constituent tasks. To '*confect*' means to make a whole by the mixture and com-pounding of ingredients. It is an organic process, with parallels in cooking. From one recipe the final product can be very different according to the art of the cook. It is not only the sum of the constituents which determines the quality of the help provided, but the way in which they are confected – the proportions, the blending, the timing and intensity of input.

All the background work that goes into the planning and provision of co-ordinated services contributes to the particular help-compact that is finally delivered to the individual user; its ultimate value depends on individual faceworkers, not only in the particular methods of help they offer but in the way these are integrated into a help-compact and the way in which the faceworker's tasks are confected during the helping process. Thus it can be said that in helping it is necessary to co-ordinate services, integrate help-compacts and confect constituent-tasks.

Non-specific methods of help often require workers to confect a number of constituents within the helping-task, and to possess flexibility and a wide range of skills. An example of such a confection follows.

The young mother

A health visitor is visiting a mother who has been failing to bring her baby to the health clinic. The helping-task, in addition to eliciting the reasons for non-attendance, might include any of the following constituent tasks: assessment of the child's health and wellbeing, practical help and teaching about feeding, information about activities at the health centre, advice about how to apply for rehousing, support for someone who is feeling inadequate. The mother's work-task, as self-helper, would include giving information and trying to convey to the health visitor the problems she is having with her child, taking advice, learning new skills, and making use of the relationship offered by the health visitor.

All the facework functions of a helping-task may be carried out by one worker but mostly they are shared with the user, as in the above case, or with other faceworkers. If the health visitor had judged it necessary to involve a doctor or a social worker, the helping-task would have been shared between them. In any event, when the mother and baby attended a clinic, a number of other workers would be providing help. When the constituents of the overall helping-task are shared between a number of faceworkers and the user, each having a particular work-task, their confection inevitably requires collaboration.

The user

It is always important to establish who is the *primary user* of the services offered. This is not always simple, as shown in the case of the schoolgirl, Clare (Chapter 2). She was the *nominated user* but not the appropriate primary user. The *user-unit* may be an individual, couple, family or a small group. Most individual users are self-helpers, and a family or group is inevitably a self-helper, since it must have strengths in order to be holding together. Where the primary user is an individual, there may well be a *concurrent user*, someone who also needs help from time to time. For example, the spouse of a person with a long-term illness may well need support and perhaps counselling, giving them the opportunity to express and come to terms with feelings which, for most people in such circumstances, are likely to be mixed. A concurrent user may be someone not actually caring for a primary user but with responsibilities towards them. For example, the adult son or daughter of a person suffering from mental illness, with a life of their own, may need help in clarifying what responsibilities for the parent they should take upon themselves.

In the case of families with dependent children it may sometimes be difficult to determine when the family and when the child is the primary user. Protecting the weak is the task of every professional and this must be a determining factor. Whilst the child is the primary user in terms of care, the family may still remain the user-unit in terms of help. Should there be serious conflict of interest between the two, the help-compact may need to be changed and the weak will take precedence as primary user.

Primary, secondary and participatory collaboration

There are times when the user cannot collaborate and is totally dependent on helpers, for example, when unconscious, totally lacking in comprehension or in a state in which rational thought is impossible. However in the majority of helping situations the user is capable of making certain decisions and carrying out certain tasks, and is in fact a potential self-helper.

When people come or are brought for help it means they have found themselves or been found in a situation where they are unable to carry total responsibility for themselves or are in need of protection. Collaboration begins when user and faceworker start working together to do something about the situation. This I call *primary collaboration*. *Secondary collaboration* describes the relationships between several helpers working together for the benefit of a user, without the latter present. *Participatory collaboration* describes the complexity of individual and group relationships that occur when the user is present and taking part, however minimally.

At the beginning of helping, it is usually possible for the faceworker to explain the help that is available and for the user to exercise some choice. In making a choice, the user shares responsibility and enters into a working relationship. Often there is only one way of bringing about betterment for the user, but that user can always exercise the negative power of refusal. At other times there may be options; for instance an elderly person no longer able to cope independently, might receive extra help and remain at home, or move into residential care. Here secondary and participatory collaboration will be necessary. In seeking any solution to a trouble there are two basic principles: first, that as a measure of wellbeing, the triple aim of helping is applied; second, that those who will share responsibility for implementing a plan, including the user as self-helper and the carer, who may well be a concurrent user, should be personally involved or represented in clarifying the options, agreeing the final plan and taking the decision to carry it out. When a help-compact needs revision, it is essential to review the balance of shared responsibility and input between user and relevant faceworker(s).

Responsibility

Taking on tasks involves responsibility, which is usually shared between user and faceworker. It is *proactive/active*, when taking initiative or control; *reactive/passive*, when stimulated by an outside source, usually a response to someone else who is taking the active part. The amount of proactive *user responsibility*, and reactive user-response, and the complementary *faceworker responsibility* and response, is often assumed without thought, but it needs to be considered, both in relation to the triple aim of helping and to the user's motivation. Motivation, the drive to achieve a particular goal, can also be proactive, when originating inside the person, or reactive when stimulated by an external impetus.

The helping relationship

A working relationship is a human relationship of a particular kind, determined and limited by the factors relevant to working together, and thus excluding many aspects of the worker's personality. A *helping relationship* is a particular kind of working relationship, between one who needs help and one who offers it, so that it has special factors which distinguish it from other kinds of working relationship. The main difference is that the purpose of the relationship is always to do something beneficial for one of the parties to it. In the case of a personal carer helping will be a component part of a more comprehensive personal relationship. For formal carers the helping relationship will be contained in a formalised working relationship, with its constraints and conditions of service, accountability to an agency and possibly also to a profession.

In looking at the primary helping relationship of formal carers I am not here concerned with the specific content of the help given to the user; this is the concern of each agency, profession or other training body. My focus is on the nature of the relationship. In this, the formation of a working alliance is fundamental. By this I mean some implicit or explicit agreement between people to work together, with at least a minimal level of trust between them. On the part of users, this means trust that the faceworker is concerned for them as an individual; on the part of faceworkers, that the user is willing to be a recipient of help and, where necessary, has some motivation to change their situation. Minimal trust between faceworkers means that whether or not they see eye to eye they are giving primacy to the wellbeing of the user. Bipartite, tripartite and group alliances are all possible.

There are four main types of relationship through which helping is carried out: caring, controlling, co-operating and collaborating. All enter into primary, secondary and participatory collaboration.

The caring relationship must be distinguished from the provision of care. Whilst care in general is a method of help, a caring relationship is a particular kind of human contact established between helper and user. It is an attitude and a feeling towards another person, which is often manifested through a specific helping-task. Everyone in a facework job needs to incorporate in their work a basic caring relationship with the user, which takes the form of respect and concern for another human being. The feelings of many helpers are stronger than this. Personal carers will have a caring relationship of varying depth and nature, according to the existing personal relationship. Very often other helpers have a relationship with the user which, whilst not going beyond the bounds of a working relationship, enhances it with caring feelings of a personal nature. Users themselves often care for their helpers, formal as well as informal, and caring enters into the relationship between helpers. *Over-care* is the negative aspect of this relationship. In the guise of care, the users' independence can be sapped and their self-responsibility diminished. This was clearly illustrated in the case of Mrs Anson, the day nursery mother (Chapter 2).

A controlling relationship is one in which power is being exercised by one person over another. This is sometimes necessary in order to provide help or protection for the benefit of users themselves, other users, or other people. The authority for such control derives either from statutory powers; professional or personal position; or conditions laid down by the agency. Control is often exercised and accepted within a collaborative relationship. Where there is open hostility a faceworker may use collaborative methods to try and form a minimal working alliance with the user. If unsuccessful, or where there is an inability to collaborate for other reasons, such as mental disorder, it may be impossible to provide help except within the framework of a strongly controlling relationship.

Over-control is the negative aspect of this relationship. The line between too much and too little control is often difficult to draw. Manipulation is a subtle form of control by which one person gets another to do what they want through an indirect use of power, whether deliberately or unwittingly. Faceworkers may manipulate users; for example, the way in which they present alternative methods of help may influence the user's choice. On the other hand, users may manipulate faceworkers by playing on their sense of duty or feelings of guilt. Faceworkers control each other, both positively and negatively, through the authorised power of their position and, on occasion through the power of their professional status or personality.

A co-operative relationship is necessary for carrying out certain methods of help. These may vary from a simple to a highly skilled activity, but require no more than routine or functional interaction and the basic caring relationship; for example the taking of X-rays. Between user and face-worker, co-operation at a superficial level can usually be assumed. However this may be undermined by underlying negative attitudes towards being helped, and by overt attitudes such as demonstrable hostility. Sometimes anxiety prevents co-operation; for example where a test is needed and the user is very nervous the technician, in order to allay anxiety, may need to relate to the user in a collaborative way, or call on the help of a nurse for this purpose.

A collaborative relationship is one where an individualised interaction between user and helper is needed. The difference might be described as that between 'operating together' and 'labouring together'; the latter making heavier demands on the people concerned. When the interaction is comparatively straightforward, I term this *simple collaboration*. *Complex collaboration* describes a situation which requires relationships of a more complicated nature, involving the attitudes and feelings of faceworkers and users. This is what can make it hard labour. Great demands may be made on those who work at the interface with users and with other faceworkers, and strong commitment and subtle skills are needed.

The outcome of certain forms of help may be largely dependent on a collaborative relationship of some depth and unless this is achieved the method will fail; for instance in certain types of counselling and psychotherapy. Some people, whether users or faceworkers, may be able to form a good co-operative or simple collaborative relationship, but may not have the capacity nor the wish to enter into a complex collaborative relationship. In this case certain methods of help are not available to them.

Co-operative and collaborative relationships can be used in unhelpful ways. *Collusion*, entered into unwittingly more often than deliberately, describes a collaborative relationship which subtly subverts the aims of the help-compact; sometimes diminishing the user's self-responsibility and maintaining an unnecessary state of dependence; sometimes diminishing the faceworkers' valid authority.

Levels of collaboration

In common usage the terms co-operation and collaboration are often interchangeable and one is assumed to include the other. When speaking generally about collaboration I follow this usage and subsume co-operation under collaboration, using the terms routine and functional collaboration as equivalents to co-operation. The levels of collaboration are therefore defined as: *routine* and *functional collaboration* or *co-operation*, *simple collaboration* and *complex collaboration*. The following hypothetical case illustrates the various levels of collaboration.

The old man

An old man who lives alone is leaving hospital after a surgical operation. He needs some short-term support and should then be able to cope on his own. To mobilise and co-ordinate the appropriate services, workers must co-operate in routine collaboration. Should the old man not achieve total independence, long-term services will be needed, with a built-in system for feedback to ensure that the help provided changes as the man's needs change. A range of faceworkers may be engaged: for example, a relative living at a distance, a neighbour, a district nurse, GP, social worker, home help, meals-on-wheels worker. Responsibilities may have to be clarified and lines of communication established, so that if, for instance, the home help or meals-on-wheels worker finds the old man in a bad condition they know whom to contact. This requires simple collaboration, the establishment of individualised contacts and lines of communication. This might be done over the phone, but the care-compact is likely to run more smoothly and be more satisfying to those involved, if there has been face-to-face contact between faceworkers.

Should doubts arise about how to ensure the old man's wellbeing, it might be necessary for some of those involved to meet with him and/or together, to assess the situation and revise the care-compact. There may be no difficulty in this, and collaboration remains simple. However, at this point, there may be differences of opinion as to the best method of care. The respective positions, attitudes and values of the user and each of the faceworkers will now be influencing their contribution to the collaborative undertaking. Inevitably their positions become more individualised, their relationships more personalised, and increased interaction is necessary in order to achieve the best outcome. Collaboration becomes complex.

As well as illustrating the different levels of collaboration this example shows how MEC (Minimum Essential Collaboration) may need to change with a changing care-compact. The example also illustrates the difference between co-ordination, integration and confection: services need to be co-ordinated; the care-compact needs to be integrated into a composite whole; and work-tasks need to be confected in an organic process.

Relational transactions

There are many relational transactions that go on within the four main modes of helping relationship. For instance, the types of exchange used when collaborating in order to reach an agreed help-compact include: communication of relevant thoughts and feelings, exploration, clarification, discussion, negotiation and bargaining. Sometimes collaboration results in a positive consensus but sometimes this cannot be achieved. If *negative consensus* – lip-service only – is not used as an evasive tactic, then a compromise will need to be sought, and bargaining may become an important process. Compromise, if carried out by open negotiation or bargaining and rooted in strong motivation, may result in an effective help-compact. In fact, it may be more firmly established and better integrated than one based on consensus, because in hammering it out clear statements of intent have been elicited from each helper, including the user as self-helper.

For consolidating agreements that have been reached and ensuring that the commitments of the user and faceworkers involved will be carried through, there are valuable *relational structures*, such as *goal-setting, task-setting*, and *contract-making*. The latter is being used increasingly, both at the managerial level and in facework collaboration. It stems from recognition of the need for clarity and control, if the helping process is to be both effective and time-efficient. At facework level a contract, usually verbal, is made concerning specific commitments. Such agreements may be made easily, others may involve negotiation and bargaining. If the latter processes uncover underlying resistances and negative feelings – whether in users or faceworkers – the contract finally reached is more likely to be fulfilled. A contract come by easily may fail because its consequences have not been thought through or because a serious commitment to it has not been made.

This completes the framework within which the collaborative relationships of faceworkers can be set. In the next two chapters I look at its application to primary, secondary and participatory collaboration.

Chapter 5
Primary Collaboration

In looking at primary collaboration I am not concerned with specific methods of practice which belong to individual professions, but with the common basis of all facework. This has two main aspects: the sharing of responsibilities between user and faceworker; and the relational input, from both user and faceworker, into the helping process.

Shared responsibility

The following example illustrates the sharing of responsibility and how it is connected with motivation.

Mrs Ingham, the stroke sufferer

Mrs Ingham, a middle-aged lady living with her teenage daughter, had suffered a severe stroke. She was making little progress in hospital, although she seemed to follow the physiotherapist's every instruction; the latter was surprised at her lack of progress. Finally the staff agreed that she would have to be transferred to permanent residential care. When told of this decision, Mrs Ingham almost immediately began to show such marked improvement that plans were delayed and in the end she was able to return home.

Having found her own motivation Mrs Ingham was able to take proactive as well as reactive responsibility for herself. A responsible attitude may be the outcome of upbringing, thought or feeling, but unless it is accompanied by an emotional drive there will be little power behind it. Users may know how they should respond to the proffered help, but until there is a wish to make something of their own lives, however conscientious the response, it will be weak. Fighting spirit is important and the strength of the user's motivation is often a determining factor in the outcome of help. Although Mrs Ingham showed a conscientious response to the instructions of the physiotherapist, there was no emotional drive. Motivation arose out of her reaction to the idea of going into residential care. She might have found proactive motivation through a collaborative relationship in which she was helped to express and work through her feelings of depression consequent to becoming physically handicapped. However, by whatever means, it was important that she found her own motivation for making the best of her life. Only then could she respond sufficiently to the physiotherapist, with whose help her condition could improve.

Responsibility for achieving the objectives of the help-compact may require the faceworker to supplement or substitute for the user's motivation. This is particularly important when users are first faced with a serious trouble by which they feel overwhelmed. The faceworker's function at this time is twofold: to stimulate reactive responsibility so that users may make use of help; and to assist them gradually to find self-motivation and take on proactive responsibility.

The degree of responsibility to be carried by a faceworker varies considerably. When issues of death or serious damage are at stake, this may necessitate taking over total responsibility and exercising constraint regardless of the wishes of either the primary or concurrent user. At the other extreme lies the controversial issue of the 'right to die' which highlights the collaborative problems that result from differing values.

Sometimes responsibilities are worked out, explicitly or implicitly, between user and helper as equals but, in most cases, it is the faceworker who has the greater influence. This may present a difficult task. For instance in mental health cases users may be able to take full responsibility for themselves at certain times, but at other times be incapable of rational thought or behaviour. Relatives and practitioners then have to decide when and how much responsibility to take.

In ordinary life it is evident that sharing responsibility requires give and take and a working out of relative positions concerning decisions and actions. This process is slower and the relationship more complex than in situations where responsibility is held by one person only. It is often quicker and easier for a worker to feed a disabled person than to help them feed themselves, or to make an assessment and propose a plan for an elderly or mentally ill person rather than help that person participate in clarifying a situation, weighing up the options and taking part in a decision. Not only does this require more time but more concern for the individual and greater skill in relational work, particularly when there may be some element of risk involved. Sharing responsibility increases the faceworker's burden of responsibility.

Power

Users, being in need of help and perhaps facing new and difficult situations, are often in a relatively weak position *vis-à-vis* faceworkers. The one who possesses what the other needs inevitably holds power. A *power-position* in the helping services derives from: the faceworker's profession which gives them competence; position in an agency which gives them access to resources and possibly certain statutory powers; and the influential power of their standing and that of their agency. Since the basis of the helping relationship is the users' lack of sufficient resources, whether material or human, to meet their own needs, there is an inevitable imbalance of power in favour of the faceworker.

At times the responsibility which a faceworker has is not matched by adequate power to discharge it. The worker may lack either the necessary skills, material resources or authority. Responsibility for this lack may be the faceworker's or it may belong higher up the line in professional training, management, policy-making or legislation. However, helpers are more often faced with the opposite situation: the need for *empowerment of the user* rather than themselves. A few practitioners are autocratic, many more exercise undue power in a benevolent paternal or maternal manner.

Health visitors' discussion

In a discussion group in which there were two health visitors, one said: 'If I make some sensible suggestion about bringing up babies, I am usually listened to when I am known to be a nurse. If people don't know, I may say exactly the same thing and nobody will take a blind bit of notice'. She added: 'It makes me realise what a lot of responsibility I have for what I say in my professional capacity'. The other health visitor went on: 'It's rather easy to give yourself a lift in this way. I have realised that sometimes quite unintentionally I have boosted my ego at the expense of a mother. I used to think that if I went into a home and found the baby crying and I picked it up and quietened it, I had done a good job. Now I realise that quite likely I did a bad job, making the mother feel deskilled while I felt so competent'.

Deskilling and *disempowerment* of the user are to be found in all professions. Nor are misuses of power confined to the faceworker. Where a person has a duty to offer help arising out of a personal or a working relationship, users have some power to control that person as a result of their right to receive help. In exercising this right, a user may try to impose on helpers responsibilities which it is not their duty to fulfil or which the user is capable of carrying for themselves. They may do it honestly or dishonestly, in order to gain access to services. In other situations, users may wittingly or unwittingly manipulate faceworkers, particularly carers, working on their feelings of concern or guilt that they are not doing enough to help. If faceworkers fall in with this, they allow users to abuse their power-position, and do them no service. In fact the first aim of helping – encouraging maximum self-responsibility – works for the benefit of the faceworker as well as the user.

Changing values are causing a reappraisal of responsibility and the use of power in many areas of professional help. Empowerment of the user has become a well-recognised objective of help. The greater the need for specialised competence for example, in cases of serious illness, the more likely are users to wish for power to be in the hands of the professional. The closer a helping situation to normal life the more natural is it for people to wish to retain power in their own hands, as is evidenced in the continuing debate over responsibilities in childbirth.

The growth of the *self-help movement* opens greater possibilities for getting help whilst retaining maximum self-responsibility. At certain times a mutual-helper may be more of a user than a helper, but at other times the situation can be reversed. In any event responsibility is shared with people in the same situation who, in terms of power-position, are felt to be nearer the same level. In most helping situations users are by definition receivers; in a self-help group, they are also in a position to offer something, possessing a certain level of competence that has been gained from personal experience. If the offer is taken up the user is on the giving end of the relationship; or perhaps in a mutual helping relationship of give and take. To be a helper means to have some power to use for good. This in itself is an enhancer of self-esteem, which in turn can increase ability to cope. Thus a positive spiral may be set going. Conversely a negative spiral can be started by a practitioner taking too much responsibility, as illustrated by Mrs Anson, the day-nursery mother (Chapter 2).

The pattern of shared responsibility may emerge differently according to the way in which it is approached and unless it starts by defining the sphere of user responsibility it may not always work out to the user's maximum benefit. It is possible for helpers to share responsibilities between them and feel well-satisfied with their work, whilst the user has been put into an unnecessarily deskilled and dependent position.

The working alliance in early stages of the help-compact

If total responsibility for the user has been assumed, the mode of relationship will be one of caring and controlling, but usually co-operative or collaborative modes are also appropriate. Many helping situations are simple, the trouble easily assessed and the answer clear, and a co-operative or simple collaborative relationship is sufficient. When the trouble is complicated a complex collaborative relationship is called for, and the mutual trust of a working alliance essential.

In the initial stage of a help-compact an early task is the collection of data, in order to define and assess the trouble. If some of the information needed is linked to feelings of distress, embarrassment or guilt, users may be afraid of breaking down, of ridicule or censure. When this is the case, a working alliance is essential to the helping-task.

Bringing out the information needed to make an assessment is a skilled function. Practitioners have some idea what information is likely to be relevant, but users may not necessarily know. Some may be afraid of taking up the worker's time with irrelevant information; others have already made their own assessment and only give the information that they have decided is relevant. In trying to collect necessary data through talking, the practitioner may find that straight questions only elicit limited answers and open questions evoke rambling digressions. A situation is needed in which the worker can guide the interview whilst enabling the user to feel free enough to say what is in their mind. This requires the establishment of both a controlling and collaborative relationship. If faceworkers do not have the skill to do this, it may be impossible for them to carry out the function of data collection adequately.

During this process the worker is also defining the type of responsibility expected of the user. This may be mainly reactive – responding appropriately to the questions of the worker. It may be a more proactive role, taking some initiative in the process of assembling relevant information and assessing the situation. What responsibility is given to the user will depend partly on the trouble presented and partly on the helping approach of the worker. In the case of Mrs Hill, the depressed single parent (Chapter 3), at first the GP had only required her passive co-operation in taking the antidepressants, but when he began to engage her in trying to understand the cause of her depression he gave her the space to take more proactive responsibility and encouraged her into a collaborative relationship.

The parents and the child psychiatrist

A much respected child psychiatrist used sometimes to begin an assessment interview by saying to the parents, words to this effect: 'You know things about your child that I cannot possibly know, and I know things about children in general that you do not know, so we have to put our heads together'.

In this way he defined the parents' responsibility as well as his own and, in the process, he was establishing a working alliance between them. Recognition of the user's as well as the worker's contribution to the helping process gives a sense of value to users, which is likely to increase self-confidence, thus helping them to contribute fully to the shared task of data collection. More than that, it helps to establish a firm foundation for continuing collaboration.

Data collection that is carried out through a collaborative process will often be an integral part of the assessment. Questions will not follow a rigid schedule but will arise out of the answers, and in such an exchange, feeling reactions and evaluative remarks will find their place. With social and psychological troubles, and with physical troubles which may have a psychogenic element, users often have an essential part to play in making a good assessment, because this can only emerge out of a collaborative exchange. A gradual process of clarification may take place so that user and faceworker will often arrive together at a joint assessment, although the final formulation may be carried out by the worker.

When giving an opinion practitioners will draw on knowledge and experience which will enable them to enlarge on the causes and likely consequences of the trouble, evaluate its seriousness and make recommendations as to possible methods of help. Users may have arrived at their own opinion, drawing on a personalised view of the situation. Through effective collaboration at the assessment and opinion-giving stages, an alignment may be achieved between the more objective views of the worker and the more subjective views of the user.

Assessment has two fundamental objectives which underlie all the others: to decide on the appropriate form of help and whether the faceworker and/ or the agency are able to provide it. This sounds straightforward, but it is complicated by the fact that the helping approach of the practitioner with whom a user first makes contact may have considerable influence on their assessment. When situations are clearly not simple and are not at a point of crisis, what is judged an appropriate assessment may vary considerably from one practitioner to another. Other determining factors are the time that is available and the user's wishes. On this basis I distinguish between the *minimum essential assessment*, *MEA* for short, and the *extended assessment*.

In making an assessment, starting at the point where the user starts, it is a question for the practitioner where and how far to go, either on their own authority or, after putting the options to the user, as a joint decision. When a practitioner considers that a presenting trouble is likely to be the manifestation of an underlying psychological, personal or social trouble, they have to decide whether it would be helpful to explore this further in order to offer more radical help rather than dealing only with the presenting trouble. Often the user, consciously or unconsciously, may be trying to cope with personal difficulties by means of the presenting trouble and may wish to avoid exploring underlying causes. Thus a marital problem may present itself in the form of frequent headaches or complaints about poor housing. Physical or practical troubles are sometimes more acceptable to the user than psychological or personal ones, the recognition of which may arouse feelings of inadequacy, shame or guilt. Whether or not the practitioner takes an integrative approach, it should be possible for them to explain the options objectively to the user. The latter may or may not welcome the opportunity to take a more radical course. It is within the practitioner's domain to give an opinion but the decision lies in the user's domain, except in exceptional circumstances.

An integrative approach, if acceptable to the user, will in many cases lead to an extended assessment, possibly requiring the participation of other workers with different skills, as in the case of Mrs Hill, the depressed single parent (Chapter 3).

In exploring underlying causes, it is often found that other helpers have already been involved, or still are, either with the same or another aspect of the user's life. With a collaborative approach, unless authority has to be exercised because the user is incapable or the situation dangerous, contacting other workers is the result of a joint decision. Where there are young children, particularly if family life is disorganised, other helpers are almost certainly already engaged. This is also true of users with a long history of psychological troubles. In such situations, an assessment which can form the basis of a comprehensive plan may only be possible if information concerning previous help is obtained and contact made with other workers. Sometimes the user may not wish for such an assessment but only seeks immediate relief from the presenting trouble. Some users may need to develop a working alliance before permitting the practitioner to contact other helpers. Some users can only take the kind of help that is offered by a drop-in centre, where they are subject to virtually no assessment. Here even the suggestion of secondary collaboration might be positively unhelpful. The need to establish primary collaboration prohibits any secondary collaboration, however desirable.

Assessing whether the user can and should be helped by the worker or agency should take into account two other options: whether the user might benefit by returning to some previous agency or worker, or going on to another one in the resource pool. For instance, someone with a psychological trouble could initially approach one of a number of agencies: a GP practice, a social services area office, health clinic, various family, counselling or drop-in centres. If any of the practitioners judged that their agency could not offer optimum help, they would assess for referral-on to another agency.

At the *planning* and *decision-making stages* of a help-compact the user's participation will depend on the nature of the trouble, the methods of help available, the practitioner's helping-approach and the user's attitude to being helped. In some situations the necessary help may be of a highly specialised or technical nature. Then it will be for practitioners to make preliminary decisions on possible options, to explain these and offer advice and recommendations to the user, who will only participate at the final decision-making stage. For some troubles there may be alternative methods which can be immediately discussed with the user. For instance, the possible help for depression, anxiety or neurotic symptoms might include drug treatment, behaviour or relational psychotherapy, family therapy, counselling, changes in social or environmental conditions. These might be offered separately or in various combinations. It will depend on the helping approach of the practitioner whether all options are presented to the user and whether the latter is helped to make their own choice. It will depend on the user's attitude how far they wish to take an active part in decision-making. Some may seek to avoid all responsibility; others, resenting their need to seek help, may seek to retain an unrealistic independence, so that they find a collaborative decision-making process extremely difficult.

The user may be actively involved in proposing as well as examining options, particularly when making long-term plans, which are often more satisfactory when arrived at through a collaborative process. The provision of the help preferred by users may not be feasible, and circumstances may force them to accept a different solution. This is likely to be more tolerable if they have taken part in the process of planning, thus being able to under-stand, step by step, why their wishes cannot be fully met. It may also make it easier to accept the situation if they have had the opportunity to express their reactions, and know that their point of view has been appreciated by workers.

The working alliance in later stages of the help-compact

In the implementation stage of a help-compact there may be specialised functions which have to be performed by practitioners or other skilled workers. Users take on many tasks, carrying out recommended treatments, looking after themselves as much as possible, making their own initiatives. It is important for faceworkers to plot the profile of a user's capabilities. Although unable to carry out many practical tasks, because of a disability, the user's capacity to plan and take decisions may be unimpaired. However, when dependent on others for practical help such decisions must be the outcome of a collaborative process. Planning the distribution of tasks is then a shared task and may well be a continuing one as the helping-process proceeds.

In the course of sharing out tasks the practitioner may have an important teaching function; but beyond acquiring new skills, the user and carer may also be learning new attitudes and ways of approaching their situation. *Modelling* is a method of help which is often unwittingly incorporated in a collaborative relationship. The practitioner provides a model with which the user or carer can identify, whether this be in the way they tackle a task or their attitude to the situation and the other people involved in it.

In methods of help based on relational work such as counselling, users always share in the task, since it is through the interactions of a collaborative relationship that the help is effected.

Many shared practical tasks which could be completed solely on a co-operative basis are carried out within a collaborative relationship which is necessary for the overall helping-task. For instance, in the rehabilitation of those who have suffered disablement skilled counselling may be of benefit over and above the support they receive. Mrs Ingham, the stroke patient might have been helped in this way. Activating proactive responsibility in users may mean allowing or enabling them to express angry or depressed feelings in order to work through them so that more positive feelings can emerge. Counselling of this kind can be used when working with user and carer together to help them share their difficult emotions and thus strengthen their working alliance. Nurses and physiotherapists can be trained to provide counselling in conjunction with physical treatments, helping the user come to terms with their feelings about being handicapped and the problems they will face on leaving hospital. This not only saves time and the introduction of a new worker but through the confection of the two methods provides a better quality of help.

Relational work that is confected with a controlling relationship may have to contain considerable resentment from the user though at a later stage the need for control may be appreciated. Collaboration does not mean that users and faceworkers always agree, nor that everything runs smoothly. In fact, where psychotherapeutic methods are being used, working on negative attitudes may be an essential part of the helping process, as was indicated in the case of Bill Bowles, the psychiatric patient (Chapter 2).

In order to strengthen user responsibility, elements of control may need to be introduced, such as goal-setting and task-setting. Within an overall plan, a short-term goal may be agreed along with the necessary tasks for user and faceworker, and sometimes contract-making is introduced with specific commitments on either side. At the end of the agreed timespan achievements are reviewed and, maybe, a new contract negotiated. Such contracts may involve negotiation and bargaining. If these processes uncover underlying resistances and negative feelings the user's proactive responsibility may be increased. Sometimes the user's commitment may be reinforced by defined rewards and penalties. In group situations such as a rehabilitation centre encouragement or censure from fellow users may be a motivating force. So long as a working alliance has been established, the processes of contract-making, goal and task-setting, although they may be felt to have a punitive element, will at a deeper level be experienced as benevolent, in a similar way to the controlling actions of good parents.

When the user is a family such relational methods can serve a dual purpose. They may help the family to become better able to cope and, at the same time, offer the parents a model for benevolent control. This was one of the aims of the child psychiatrist with the Foster family (Chapter 2). He used his professional authority to help the parents find ways of exercising their parental authority more firmly; at the same time he discussed with the whole family sensible ways in which this should be carried out, so that the children might participate in a contract-making process. By contrast the approach of the GP was to accept the proffered authority and give advice, despite the fact that he had a working alliance with the mother which could have been used to encourage self-responsibility rather than dependency.

The place of feeling in the helping relationship

In all helping situations the basic caring relationship must be present and its importance to the user cannot be overestimated. Interaction with another person, even of the most superficial or fleeting kind, may involve the feelings of one or both people. In a co-operative task, where feelings are not intrinsically relevant to the task, each person will handle his or hers in their own way; in collaborative tasks, some of the feelings of both user and faceworker will be relevant. This is not the place to discuss methods of help like psychotherapy which specifically involve working on relationships. However as regards the helping relationship itself, in the process of receiving various kinds of help it may be essential for users to feel that they are understood, their situation appreciated, and they themselves valued. They may not need counselling; just someone with whom they feel they can share their distress without being too much of a burden. This applies as much, if not more, to concurrent users as to primary users.

Mrs Knight, carer

> **M**rs Knight, describing how she had looked after her husband at home when he was terminally ill with cancer, said: 'One day I was in our corner shop, and an acquaintance asked me how my husband was. I just burst into tears. The lady who ran the shop took me upstairs and gave me a cup of tea. She had to go down again, but she was kind and I was so relieved to be able to sit there and not have to stop crying. When she came up again, we only spoke a few words, but she was such a comfort to me. I felt able to go back into my house. You see I couldn't let myself cry in the house for fear I should not be able to stop, and it would have upset him too much to see me so upset'.

In offering emotional as well as practical support to personal carers, neighbours are a great strength. The weakening of neighbourhood cohesion and neighbourliness has led to a diminution of help from the community so that a greater obligation falls on the formal carers to take care of the feelings of carers. Although responding appropriately to the user's feelings can hardly be deemed a specific method of help in itself, it is an essential component of methods of support.

One of the strengths of self-help groups is the mutual support of feeling understood and valued. Members are also likely to trust others who are, or have been, 'in the same boat'. In some ways mutual helpers may be less trustworthy than the professionals, who are strengthened by their ethical code and accountability; but this is outweighed by the importance of fellow-feeling. The shared trouble gives a user an experience of belonging somewhere, a stronger and more positive sense of identity and greater personal value. Perhaps it is because these are imponderable factors that they have not been given sufficient weight in some approaches to helping.

The user's concern for the feelings of faceworkers depends on whether the latter are formal or informal carers. To be concerned for the feelings of the formal carer is not an essential part of the primary user's responsibility, whereas, wherever possible, with the informal carer it is. If the helping-task is prolonged and stressful, feelings on both sides may become difficult to manage, and a process of working through the difficulties together with the assistance of a third person may help the personal relationship and maintain the quality of life of both people.

The faceworker's personal involvement

This has three aspects: personal information, personal style, and involvement of the helper's feelings. The amount of personal detail which is communicated to the user and the informality of the helper's personal style are partly an individual matter, but are often inversely correlated to the degree of professionalisation of the job. They may also be related to the particular help-method and setting, and the type of relationship which has developed between user and helper, its depth and duration. Variations between one worker and another are unimportant compared with the need for consistency in the individual faceworker, so that the user knows what to expect. Along with changes in society the style of helping relationships is becoming freer. However the carrying out of certain helping tasks is made easier for both user and practitioner when a formal relationship is maintained since this can contain difficult emotions which cannot be coped with at the time. In all stressful situations it benefits users if at least one of the helpers can show that they appreciate their feelings. In many situations more is required. Then the faceworker needs the capacity to give an individualised feeling response. For practitioners this is not the same as a personal response because limits to their personal involvement are set through containment in their particular helping-role. How the practitioner's emotions are contained and controlled is a matter of great significance in helping, and will be discussed in Chapter 11.

I have given an example in the case of Clare Cooke, the symptomatic schoolgirl (Chapter 2), of how the unwitting input of users can involve, in a mirroring process, the behaviour and feelings of practitioners. Another process in which faceworkers become unwittingly involved originates within themselves in response to the user's situation. This is the process of *emotional identification*, which is illustrated in the following example.

Jimmy Johnson and his mother

Mrs Johnson's little boy of four, had been referred by the paediatrician to the child psychiatrist; his IQ was a little below average and his behaviour very difficult. Mrs Johnson described Jimmy as very overactive, never settling to anything, always round her, so that she could not get on with things. He was getting worse and she felt at the end of her tether. He became a little quieter when her husband came in; only then, when she was exhausted, did she complete her housework, before getting a meal and putting Jimmy to bed. He was their only child and she felt she could not have another because she would have neither time nor energy to look after a second one properly. They had always intended to have a bigger family as they were both fond of children. The psychiatrist suggested that she should bring Jimmy to the hospital for regular appointments with a child therapist whilst she talked with the social worker, to see if they could work out ways of managing Jimmy. She said that Jimmy was such a handful on a bus that she could not do this, although she would have liked to. It was then arranged that the social worker would visit her at home.

Mrs Johnson welcomed the social worker and they began talking, whilst Jimmy clambered round them. The social worker tried to engage him in conversation and to settle him with some of his toys, but without much success. Mrs Johnson said: 'I am glad you have come, because you can see just what he is like. I sometimes feel people won't believe me', and she broke down in tears. She poured out her distress, the accumulation of years of difficulty and loneliness. She said that, although she had a good husband, he did not seem able to listen when she tried to tell him how she felt and just told her that she was doing very well and that it would be better when Jimmy got to school age. She did not know whether the school would take him; the future seemed hopeless. Whilst Mrs Johnson unburdened herself, the social worker did not interrupt, but began to feel utterly hopeless herself. Jimmy stood still, watching his mother intently.

When the social worker saw the psychiatrist next morning, she immediately spoke to him about Mrs Johnson, saying she felt she could not go on with the case because she felt so utterly hopeless about it. He was surprised, saying that she had never before suggested giving up a case like that, and asked what had happened. She said that while with Mrs Johnson she had felt very strongly that she must make things better for this mother but quite unable to do so. Now, looking back and seeing again the expression on Jimmy's face, as he stood there, she thought that he must have been feeling like that. She said: 'I wish now that I had said something to him about how worried he must sometimes feel about his mother'.

After further discussion, the psychiatrist suggested that the next appointment should be at the hospital and that they should see Mrs Johnson and Jimmy together, hoping that she would manage to bring him. She did come, looking very different and saying that she felt better able to cope after having talked with the social worker.

It seems that the social worker had been able to help Mrs Johnson but in the process had internalised emotions that currently were not hers. Another faceworker might have been able to help as much, without suffering in the same way. Different people are vulnerable to different situations, according to their personality and past. My purpose here is not to go deeply into the practice of relational work, but to outline the aspects of the helping relationship which are common to all faceworkers, one of which is emotional identification. Mrs Johnson's case is not an unusual one. It demonstrates the kind of emotional complexity that can arise in primary collaboration. Here the practitioner was a social worker, but faceworkers of any profession and those who are not trained, may be caught up in this process of emotional identification. It poses a problem for faceworkers in being in touch with the feelings of users without being overburdened by them.

Those who attempt relational work with disturbed or socially disorganised families are particularly vulnerable to the process of emotional identification, sometimes experiencing feelings of guilt or anger as well as responsibility and failure. The needs of such families often require considerable secondary collaboration, and if faceworkers have become caught in this process it will inevitably affect their relationships with other workers as well as the user.

The common factors in all helping relationships

The two most important aspects of primary collaboration common to all faceworkers lie in the areas of responsibility and feeling. In complex collaboration, shared responsibility, whether for tasks or for decision-making, emerges as a key concept. Matters of feeling lend themselves less easily to conceptualisation. In earlier examples and those in this chapter I have tried to show the subtle nature of feelings in helping relationships and how they may have an important influence on the outcome of help. However, underlying all the emotional complications of complex collaboration, the basic emotion needed by a faceworker is that of fellow-feeling which almost inevitably leads to a caring attitude. It can be said that shared responsibility and a caring attitude are the twin foundations of primary collaboration.

Chapter 6
Secondary and Participatory Collaboration

Two of the main purposes of secondary collaboration between two or more faceworkers are: to provide an integrated help-compact for a particular user through co-ordinating services and integrating methods; and to provide the kind of help which can only be achieved where there is interactive work between the faceworkers involved. Participatory collaboration takes place when the user works with more than one faceworker at the same time. This may be directly, when the user, as self-helper, participates in a meeting with two or more faceworkers; or indirectly when, although only meeting with one faceworker at a time, the self-helper is part of an interactive pattern of relationships involving a number of helpers. I give four examples to illustrate some of the processes of secondary and participatory collaboration.

Secondary collaboration

The following example shows a change from parallel help to collaborative interaction.

Len Leigh, the landscape gardener

A local mental health association was running a work project to landscape and plant a garden, as part of a community plan for developing a derelict site. The people employed had psychiatric troubles, and some were attending the local psychiatric unit. One of the main aims of the project was to help users become more responsible for themselves. The project leader was not totally averse to medication but did not see it as the answer to the users' troubles. When they started work she did not contact their psychiatrist.

Len Leigh was keen to reduce his drugs and began to do so on his own initiative, telling the project worker what he was doing. His moods became more difficult and she was worried about him, but she did not wish to diminish his self-responsibility. Sharing her worries with colleagues, she realised that Len seemed to need his two helpers to collaborate and was subconsciously trying to engineer it, but still she did not want to take on more responsibility for him. The result was that she encouraged Len to seek an early appointment with the psychiatrist. Before he went, she discussed with Len the possibility of

61

the three of them working together, to see if he could achieve his aim of reducing the medication. If Len wished, he could ask the psychiatrist to contact her. The psychiatrist did so and over the phone they established a working alliance. Len was happy for the project leader to take on a monitoring role, reporting to the psychiatrist on the effects of changes in his prescription. Here the user himself linked up the two workers who were providing concurrent help. Len's level of self-esteem was raised by having been judged capable of taking this responsibility, and the fact that he had exercised some power in initiating the collaboration between the two workers increased his trust in them. He said when he was talking in the project's discussion group about what had happened that he did not mind them discussing his progress without his knowing just what they were saying about him. This had an influence not only on the attitudes of other users but also on those of the project leader.

She arranged to meet with some of the psychiatrists in the hospital and established a good general understanding with them, although their views on mental health diverged from hers in many respects. The pattern was established in which users working in the project knew that they could initiate specific links between their psychiatrist and the project leader.

The shape that secondary collaboration takes in any particular case is influenced by the helping approach of the various faceworkers. Here it becomes clear that it need not matter if these do not coincide, so long as a working alliance can be established with agreement on the particular form of collaboration.

If users have a well-integrated personality they can probably take what they need from the practitioners and not be too concerned whether the views of the latter conflict. However need for help often stems from lack of personal or family integration. Then users are likely to be dependent on the practitioners and, finding them in conflict – as in the case of the Foster family and their smoking teenagers (Chapter 2) – may be put under added strain, and receive less effective help. Practitioners used to working independently may not be alert to the need for interactive work. In Len Leigh's case the project worker was not a practitioner. Her flair, initiative and helping approach made her a valuable project worker but did not dispose her to link up with established practitioners. It was the user who had to show her the need for such collaboration.

Frequently, problems arising from lack of collaboration are not so great as to become obvious, although they are great enough to reduce the value of the help given. This is illustrated in the following example, which came to light fortuitously.

Melvin Manson, and his three helpers

At an inter-agency meeting designed to discuss general matters of collaboration, a particular user was mentioned and became the focus of discussion.

The case was well-known to three workers present – a probation officer, a GP and a worker in a local residential therapeutic community. The purpose of this unit was to help its members, in the group and individually, to understand and modify the personal and relational problems which were hampering them in life. It emerged that all three faceworkers assumed they were the 'key worker' and also assumed this was understood by the others. When the young man, Melvin Manson, had entered the residential therapeutic community, all three had co-ordinated the help they were providing. The probation officer, as well as sending reports, had had personal contact with the head of the unit and they had arranged that Melvin should continue to visit him at certain intervals. The GP had written concerning the long medical history and the medication he was pre-scribing, for which Melvin would continue to come to him. He assumed he was the 'key worker' because there was a long history of physical and mental ill-health; further, he had known Melvin since boyhood and had sometimes given him fatherly advice, as he lived alone with his mother. The probation officer assumed that he was the 'key worker' because he had a special authority from the court, had been instrumental in arranging the residential placement, was still seeing Melvin occasionally and visiting his mother. The residential worker assumed she was the 'key worker', being in the closest relationship with the user and helping him with his personal difficulties. All three were surprised that the others took a different view from themselves, and appeared to feel that their input was not fully appreciated.

The residential worker asked the GP if he had ever visited the unit. He had not; he had heard about it from Melvin, and now perhaps it would be a good idea if she explained more about their methods. He sounded critical and in the ensuing discussion it emerged that he had built up a different picture of the place from talking to Melvin. The latter, when he came for his prescrip-tion, often spoke negatively about the community, in particular this worker, complaining that he did not get sufficient help and saying that she was like his mother. The GP had listened sympathetically. He had never thought of con-tacting the unit. He thought they should have known from his initial report that he had a special relationship with the family, and it was for the unit head to contact him. The residential worker was critical of the GP, pointing out that he encouraged Melvin to split his helpers into good and bad figures, and this would not help him. The GP replied that the residential worker did not appreciate the importance of his longstanding relationship with Melvin. He was not going to jeopardise this by refusing to discuss the residential unit with him. The probation officer explained to the GP that, whilst this long-term relationship was of the greatest importance to Melvin, the main help at the moment was coming from the residential unit and that Melvin should be encouraged to express his negative feelings there rather than elsewhere. He, as probation officer, followed this line, taking a low profile himself for the time being. The GP commented that it was difficult, when so many people were trying to help one person and nobody seemed to be in charge. The probation officer replied that he supposed if anybody were in charge he was.

Separatist attitudes

What is evident in Melvin's case is failure to see the kind of collaboration that was necessary following an important change in the help-compact. As the helping process develops or as new factors come into the situation an existing help-compact will need to be reshaped. Whenever there is a transitional stage from one help-method to another, particularly if a change of setting is involved, it is important to consider what steps are necessary to reintegrate the help-compact. Here, relevant communication, probably requiring a meeting, could have prevented the present fragmented situation. The meeting could have been initiated by the unit head or the probation officer, who were jointly responsible for the new situation. Fragmentation was aggravated by the restricted viewing-point of the unit worker and the GP. Neither fully appreciated that their input was only part of a total help-compact, which had breadth and length extending beyond the limits of their particular help. The importance of the work within the therapeutic community had caused its worker to underestimate the significance of the rest of the user's life, with which she was not personally involved; this included the time before and after his stay in the residential setting and the time he was currently spending outside it. The GP had not appreciated the significance of the user's changed circumstances, the currently important authority role of the probation officer and therapeutic role of the unit worker. The probation officer, although taking a more comprehensive view of the situation, either was unaware of or underestimated the long-term relationship the user had with his GP. A busy practitioner may well react to the stereotype of another profession. In this part of London the GP stereotype was of a doctor who took little personal interest in his patients, and the GP in this case was exceptional. Had the probation officer realised this, he might have worked more closely with him and encouraged the unit worker to do the same. In the long term, whilst probation would come to an end, the GP's help would continue.

Here we see the effects of a restricted viewing-point militating against an integrative approach to the user. It stems from ignorance about other professions and agencies, and lack of awareness of the need to confect work-tasks. Such narrow vision almost always causes the contribution of other helpers to be undervalued. In such a situation, when faceworkers come to face each other instead of the user, the place for collaborative interaction may well be filled by rivalry.

Where faceworkers are in relationship over a number of cases, they have the opportunity to form an alliance which is better able to cope with rivalry, through developing something of a team approach to their work. This can only happen over time. To achieve a working alliance specifically for one case is much more difficult, and only occasionally can the expenditure of time be spread over other cases. However, in many situations, unless faceworkers have a common understanding of the situation as a whole and the interconnection of their individual parts within it, the value of the help-compact to which they are all contributing will be diminished. In the case of Melvin we see how the opportunity for splitting his helpers into good and bad figures was detracting from the unit's efforts to help him cope with life more adequately. Repeating patterns were present. His difficulties in becoming independent of his mother were appropriately transferred on to the residential worker, where they could be discussed and understood, thus helping him to find new ways of coping. But he also involved the GP, who identified with Melvin's negative feelings and, without checking first, condoned them rather than helped him to deal actively with the situation. When the GP met the unit worker he brought these feelings into the group discussion, but an earlier meeting might have avoided such a situation ever developing.

Interactive work

If workers are to provide optimal help where repeating patterns or mirroring processes are operating, it is essential that they communicate their attitudes and feelings both about the user's situation and each other's input into the help-compact. Whether or not users are physically present, they are often effectively there, and influencing the faceworkers. Processes go on in secondary collaboration which are not always easily explained, and this is particularly true when feelings are strong in a group meeting. The presence and nature of repeating patterns and mirroring processes can only be identified if workers are able to communicate openly.

There is usually something in the worker which is ready to pick up the particular feelings of the user. In the case of Mrs Gould (Chapter 2), the education welfare officer's mistrustful attitudes towards psychiatry in general and to the local child psychiatric department and its social worker in particular, may have been entirely his own. However, their strength and the way in which he acted on them in face of a group decision, suggest that there may have been a mirroring process at work: that, without realising it, he may have taken on some of Mrs Gould's strong feelings about the situation. In doing so he would make it easy for her to avoid expressing them herself to the worker concerned. This would remove the opportunity for Mrs Gould to test out her feelings in a relationship with the social worker, which might have helped her to manage, if not modify, her negative attitudes to receiving psychiatric help. Later she did, in fact, make a more trusting relationship with the social worker and eventually began to attend a psychiatric day centre.

For faceworkers to internalise the feelings, relational patterns and attitudes of users is such a common phenomenon that to find ways of either neutralising or making good use of this process is essential. If feelings can be voiced in a group, they can be responded to openly, as in Melvin's case. If, as a result, faceworkers gain increased understanding this can be used in the process of helping the user. If the GP understood the situation well enough, when he next saw Melvin he could take the line that, although there might well be things wrong with the unit, it was not for the two of them to discuss these matters but for Melvin to bring up his grievances in the unit. As a GP who knew the family situation very well, he might possibly have drawn a parallel between Melvin's current complaints and those he was wont to make about his mother.

Where the user is a family, it is common, during a group discussion, for faceworkers to identify with different members of it. If expression of relevant feelings is open, the recognition of this process often results in greater understanding of relationships and tensions within the family.

Mrs Newman, would-be adoptive mother

A mother, Mrs Newman, took her youngest child Helen, aged eight, to the GP, because of loss of appetite. From time to time, when small, she had gone off her food but never for as long as this. The GP gave a prescription, reassured Mrs Newman and suggested that, if the symptoms did not clear up in a fortnight, they should visit him again. They did return and on this occasion he went into the matter more thoroughly. He came to the conclusion that there must be some emotional problem which Helen did not bring out and neither he nor her mother could identify. He suggested referral to a child psychiatric clinic, which Mrs Newman accepted. The clinic invited both parents to come with all their children. Three of these appeared lively and healthy and one looked pale and depressed. It turned out that this was not Helen but a little girl, Pam, whom the Newmans had been looking after for some weeks, and whom she had not mentioned to the GP.

In this meeting and a subsequent one with the clinic social worker the following story emerged: Mr Newman kept a pub, which Pam's mother had frequented. She was a vulnerable young woman, drinking and smoking too much, appearing to have neither family nor friends and living alone with her daughter. Pam and Helen were school friends and Helen often brought Pam home for tea. Mrs Newman incorporated her into the family as much as possible and Pam's mother was grateful. Quite unexpectedly, the latter died. Mrs Newman offered to look after Pam, and the area social worker accepted this as a temporary measure while she worked out a long-term plan. Mrs Newman secretly hoped to adopt Pam, although she did not mention this to her husband or the area social worker. In the interview, Mrs Newman then broke down and told the clinic social worker that some years ago she had become pregnant and, for health reasons, had been strongly advised to have a termination. Her husband was in favour but she was against it, on religious grounds. However, the priest said if her health and her ability to care for her existing three children was seriously jeopardised by the pregnancy, termination would not be wrong. After the termination, she felt very distressed but did not speak of this to her husband, GP or priest, saying that she knew they were right and she was being silly. She often thought of the lost baby, and in providing a home for Pam felt she could do something to make amends.

In a further meeting, Mrs Newman told the clinic worker that an aunt of Pam's mother had been traced and was ready to give Pam a permanent home. She was married with grown-up children, and the area social worker thought her a suitable person. Having found it impossible to help or get near her niece, she had scarcely ever met Pam, but had worried about her and was glad to take care of her. Mrs Newman was very distressed. She was convinced that the great-aunt was taking Pam for the wrong reasons, out of a sense of duty, and would never be able to love her enough. She felt it was dreadful to send Pam to someone she did not know, to a new school and away from all her friends. The clinic social worker suggested contacting the area social worker, and got the mother's consent to mention the termination, if the occasion should arise.

The clinic worker arranged a meeting with the GP, area social worker and the senior social worker involved. The latter said she had interviewed and liked the great-aunt, had visited her home, met the great-uncle and, as they were blood relations and caring people, she thought this was a good permanent home for Pam. In the discussion, the clinic social worker expressed doubts about this decision, voicing some of Mrs Newman's arguments against it. The GP was convinced that Pam should leave the family, because he thought her presence there was the cause of Helen's trouble. The area social worker, who had let her senior do all the talking, suddenly said, with considerable feeling, that Pam had never been consulted and would probably prefer to stay where she was. This brought the mounting tension in the group to a climax. The succeeding discussion took a new turn. All four workers began to realise that they were speaking as a protagonist for one of the people in the situation, and the two most involved began to de-identify themselves. The clinic social worker's feelings began to change and she said that in fact she did trust the senior social worker's judgement. The area social worker said she knew that Pam was too young to make the decision herself about her future.

The final phase of the discussion was characterised by a shared determination to ensure that the feelings of each of the people involved should be properly appreciated and cared for while the plan was being implemented. The clinic social worker would continue to work with Mrs Newman, helping with her feelings about the termination and Pam's departure, two closely related losses, and so perhaps enable her to withdraw some of her negative feelings from the great-aunt. The area social worker would explain the decision to Pam and, in as far as was possible at this time, help her with her reactions. Both primary faceworkers now felt unhampered by doubts about the plan. The senior social worker would use her increased understanding of the situation to enable Mrs Newman and the great-aunt to get to know each other and work together to achieve Pam's move in an atmosphere of goodwill. The GP, who would be monitoring Helen's health, was now aware of the situation and Mrs Newman's distress.

The value of interactive work illustrated here has several aspects. First, although the main decisions taken in these two overlapping cases would probably have been the same whether or not the workers had met, their implementation was different in important respects. Second, the quality of help given would not have been possible without the meeting, in which the mirroring process was able to manifest. By expressing their feelings, the two involved faceworkers enabled the group to play out between them the troubled situation with which they were trying to grapple. Once recognised, the mirroring by the clinic social worker of Mrs Newman's attitudes, and the emotional identification of the area social worker with Pam were turned to good advantage in planning the help-compact instead of operating negatively. Third, two separate situations needing help overlapped – Pam's need to be settled in the right home on a long-term basis, and Mrs Newman's need for counselling as a result of her termination – and the optimal solution for each of them could only be achieved through the workers entering into a collaborative process. The optimum for Pam depended on her moving to her great-aunt in a way which would not be unnecessarily stressful nor would sever the meaningful relationships of her past life. This could easily have happened, as a result of tension between the two mother substitutes caused by Mrs Newman's hostility to the great-aunt. The optimum for Mrs Newman depended on her being able to work with the great-aunt to help Pam in this way and, at the same time to disentangle her feelings for this child from those for her lost baby. Fourth, the MEC required for optimal help in the two cases was that of the four practitioners and one meeting. The meeting was time-efficient; the expenditure of approximately eight man-hours was justified in terms of the resulting quality of help given to those badly needing it. Fifth, the long-term cost-benefit can be postulated although it cannot be proven. It could be that without the counselling which Mrs Newman received at this time – working to sort out the linked situations of Pam and the termination – she might have become more depressed and irritable, with possible harmful effect on her children as well as herself; she might well have needed a greater amount of help for herself later in life. It could be that if Pam's move had not been well managed, so that the break was not too traumatic, it would have been more difficult for this very vulnerable child to settle in her new home; thus adding to her vulnerability in the future. Who knows? The value of preventive work is rarely quantifiable.

Participatory collaboration

Even if workers have developed satisfactory methods of secondary collaboration, it is not easy to enter into participatory work. This requires the adaptation of established patterns of practitioner-user relationships. If a worker has been used to meeting with users by themselves and in their own agency, to meet with them in another setting and in a group with other workers brings up new relational problems. The following example illustrates some of the difficulties.

Oliver Ogden, aggressive adolescent

A teenage boy, Oliver Ogden, had been excluded from school, following repeated bouts of dangerously violent behaviour. An area social worker had been working with him and his family, and had arranged for them to be seen by the psychiatrist at the child guidance clinic. The conclusion was reached that Oliver had a personality disturbance which would best be helped by admission to the regional adolescent unit. The headmaster agreed. The psychiatrist in charge of the unit, before admitting someone of school age who would probably return home and reattend his previous school, liked to have a meeting with the headteacher and other professionals involved, followed immediately by all of them meeting the parents and the young person. The aim was to establish the stay in the unit as part of a continuous helping process.

The meeting was held in the area social work office, the first part attended by the unit's psychiatrist and social worker who would be in contact with the parents while the boy was in the unit, headmaster and area social worker. They were all in agreement about the proposed plan. Then they were joined by Oliver and his mother, who said that Mr Ogden was unable to be present, being a long-distance lorry driver. The psychiatrist took charge of the meeting, explaining the kind of help that was offered in his unit, its daily routine, the reasons for Oliver going there and how it might help him. He and his mother were then encouraged to participate in the discussion, which covered the fear of mental illness and the stigma of a psychiatric label. Mrs Ogden voiced her worries about her son's behaviour and the fact that his father was away such a lot. She had had to rely on the school to provide the discipline that Oliver needed and she felt they had been very helpful to him. The headmaster said that his teachers liked Oliver and spoke well of him, except for the violent outbursts, but these had become too much for the school to contain. The boy then joined in, saying that on the last occasion he had felt it was unfair that he had been excluded from school and not some of the other boys who had also been behaving badly. The head explained why he had done this. The psychiatrist then enlarged on how admission to the unit was not a punishment but a way of trying to help. The head seemed rather withdrawn during this discussion, until there was a pause, when he entered the conversation, saying that he had been thinking that perhaps he should take Oliver back into school. He turned to the boy and asked whether he thought he could control his temper if given one more chance. Oliver looked pleased and said he would try, and Mrs Ogden said she would do her best to keep him up to it. They left soon after this, but the professionals continued their discussion.

The psychiatrist was annoyed at the headmaster's turnabout. The latter apologised and found it difficult to explain what had made him change his mind. He said that if he had been interviewing the boy and his mother on their own in his study, he would probably have held to the decision, but being in this meeting, where he was not in charge, and watching their distress, he had begun to question his previous decision.

They continued to discuss the future of Oliver, and the need to provide him with some special help for his violent outbursts. They headmaster said that he would discuss this with the boy's tutor and the local child guidance clinic. He thought he would make attendance there a condition of Oliver being accepted back into school. He would not make it a condition that the parents attended but it might be that they needed help too and could get it there.

We do not know whether or not the outcome of this meeting was in the best interests of Oliver. What can be clearly seen is the unexpected and subtle factors that influence workers when entering into participatory collaboration. The relationship of a professional worker to an individual or family user is based on training and experience, and the balance of power is weighted on the side of the professional. An interview usually follows well-tried patterns as does that between professionals. When practitioners jointly meet the user, these familiar patterns are superseded by a group situation containing both user and colleague relationships. Each worker may be reacting concurrently to the user and to some or all of the other workers in a complicated pattern of interweaving relationships. They may be influenced by such things as the location of a meeting – it is not on their territory; their power-position – they are not in charge of the meeting; some or all of the participants may be unknown to them; they may find that the participant users, whom they already know, behave and contribute differently with other workers; they have a greater opportunity to be an observer.

We do not know what caused the headmaster to change his mind. From comments made in other groups there is evidence that, because of rivalry, practitioners often do not find it easy to accept that other professionals have skills to help where their own skills have failed. But the head may have been quite right to change his mind, as a result of the process that went on in this group.

The meeting failed to achieve its declared objective but, in terms of the ultimate wellbeing of the boy, it may have been successful. Time may not have been wasted, if it meant that Oliver was able to remain in school and go to an out-centre for psychotherapeutic help. Equally, if his behaviour failed to improve and later he went to the residential unit, the meeting might have been a valuable part of the helping process, because of its importance to Oliver. He might enter the unit with a different attitude, knowing that his earlier feelings about being treated unfairly had been heard and appreciated. With the further experience at school, he might be able to accept his need for help with his violent emotions and therefore be in a better position to make use of it. In helping it is not always possible to know what is helpful.

What emerges from this and the previous example is, first, the importance of practitioners listening to, and appreciating, the feelings of users; and, second, how this makes practitioners more vulnerable. In both these cases the users' feelings had a considerable influence on the practitioners, whose vulnerability led to a humanised response. The process demanded professional integrity and the effort to combine subjective reactions with objective judgement.

Even when there is a well-established relationship between faceworkers, the presence of a user can cause difficulties when it puts them in an unfamiliar position.

Mr Quinn, referring on

In a meeting of a group for mental health workers, a social worker from a drop-in centre and one from a counselling agency together described the difficulties they had experienced over a recent referral. Mr Quinn had consulted the drop-in worker about his personal problems, and she had thought that he could use the help of the counselling agency. She phoned the agency and, in the man's presence, spoke to a worker whom she knew well. She was asked some questions by the counsellor about her assessment of Mr Quinn's troubles and his motivation, which she found difficult to answer adequately while he was listening. The counsellor became irritable at her vague replies and her apparent wish for him to accept the case on her recommendation. Finally, she said that he had better talk to Mr Quinn himself and handed over the phone. In presenting his side of the situation, the counsellor said that as soon as he was talking directly with Mr Quinn, he felt sure how to proceed, treating it as a self-referral and, after a short discussion, making an appointment to see him. The counsellor said he had felt angry with the drop-in worker for apparently trying to make a decision for him. She said that if she had been on her own, she would have answered all his questions and he could have made his own decision. As it was, she felt she could not talk as one practitioner to another with the man sitting there. Knowing the agency so well, she had been sure it was a case for them. He replied that he still liked to make his own decision, adding: 'and why shouldn't the man have presented his own case?' She agreed that he was quite capable of doing so, but it had not occurred to her; on reflection, perhaps she had tried to be too helpful.

Questions were raised as to whether practitioners sought sanction from users to speak for them; whether users were encouraged and enabled to do this for themselves; the terms in which practitioners couched their opinions, when the user was present; on what occasions practitioners should and should not involve users in their discussions. One worker suggested that a good basis for deciding such questions might be what she would feel in the user's position. Someone said that it was unlikely that this worker would be in such a disturbed state as some of her clients. She replied that she was not so sure. Another said that people were not all the same; some wanted to be involved, others might prefer not to know what the practitioners were saying about them. Perhaps users should be participating in the decision about when they should or should not take part in discussions about themselves.

The issue raised above is one of considerable importance to participatory collaboration. What is the nature of the boundary overlap between helper and user when it comes to describing the latter's situation? How much does this vary according to the user's trouble, intelligence, education, cultural background, gender, personality type, etc.?

The above example also highlights the need to distinguish between the case and the user. The counsellor on one end of the phone was trying to hold a case discussion, in order to decide whether the case was suitable for his agency. On the other end of the phone, the drop-in worker was involved in a participatory discussion. The two processes were found to be incompatible.

There are times when it is necessary for practitioners to discuss a user's situation as a case, in order to reach as objective an opinion as possible about its nature and what help could be offered by themselves or others. They may need to sort out their various domains and their possible identifications, as in the case of Mrs Newman, the would-be adoptive mother. These processes would be hindered by having to take account of the user's personal feelings. There are other times when user-participation is essential to the optimal outcome of a helping process. In many situations it is not clearcut whether or not to involve a user. Sometimes the two kinds of meeting are needed in close succession.

In coming to a conclusion, two important criteria are the user's wishes and the practitioners' judgement concerning the main purpose of the meeting and the effect of participation on the user and on the outcome of help. The judgement of practitioners will be influenced by their past practice, whether or not they value a participatory approach and their ability and willingness to cope with the kind of relational problems between practitioners that participatory collaboration is likely to cause. These problems will become clearer and some may be avoided, as participatory practice develops.

When to call a meeting and who should expend time on it raises various questions. Unless formalised guidelines have been laid down, as in certain child care situations, the initiative for calling a meeting may be taken by one or another worker involved in a case.

Whose meeting?

In a small group discussion in a psychiatric hospital, the case was presented of a disturbed woman who drank heavily and had at one time belonged to Alcoholics Anonymous. She had been admitted some time ago but had discharged herself. She had been difficult about taking medication and had not kept her out-patient appointment. There were two children, who could be at risk emotionally, and an area social worker was involved, although the children were not on the at-risk register. The psychiatrist had talked on the phone with her. Recently the woman's husband had contacted the hospital, asking for a further admission. The psychiatrist was uncertain whether the woman would agree to readmission and whether it would help her; there were no grounds for compulsory admission. The group thought that he should set up a meeting to include the social worker, the woman and her husband. The psychiatrist was unenthusiastic about taking on the task. It would take time, and the patient had already taken up a good deal of his time to no effect. Other of his cases had higher priority. In the discussion that followed, the group decided that it was for the social worker to call the meeting, because she carried the greatest responsibility for the family. The psychiatrist was prepared to phone her and make this suggestion. He said that he thought the hospital the most appropriate place to hold the meeting, because the main problem was, after all, the woman's mental state. Someone asked: 'Does that mean you would chair the meeting?'

This discussion shows how the task of calling a meeting is likely to fall to the faceworker in the case who feels the greatest sense of responsibility. To arrange a meeting is a laborious task which a secretary cannot usually undertake, because those approached need to be put in the picture and may wish to discuss the reasons for their attendance. In the psychiatrist's response we have an illustration of two aspects of responsibility. The work involved in taking primary responsibility is sometimes undesired and, if possible, passed on; at other times it is desired, since it is an acknowledgement of professional position. The venue for a meeting is always significant. It is an important factor in establishing *professional primacy*; it saves travelling time; it may affect the choice of chairperson, which gives status and reinforces primacy.

In a group of four people there would in fact be no need for a formal chairperson, but there would be a need for one of the practitioners to have informal charge of the meeting, setting the objectives and ensuring that they were fulfilled. The position of each practitioner in the above example would be very different, according to the venue of the meeting and the carrier of the informal chairing role. The process of the meeting might also be different, though this would depend more on the helping approach, rather than profession, of the chairperson. What is apparent here is that, where there are no formal structures or guidelines, the no-man's land may either be left unattended or may easily become a battleground.

Chapter 7
Facework Structures and the Resource Pool: Collaborative Framework II

Complex collaboration can take a great deal of time, and maximum value out of any collaborative enterprise is achieved through applying the principle of MEC, that is the minimum number of people with the necessary level of competence using the minimum amount of their time. This requires effective facework structures and a wide viewing-point when considering resources. Here I set out a framework within which to consider collaborative practice.

Facework procedures

These are designed to order relationships, particularly in reference to authority, responsibility and tasks. *Referrals* are of two kinds – *referring on* for *sequential work* and *concurrent* referral for the introduction of additional help. In both, the working relationships between user, referring and receiving faceworkers and the *transitional work* carried out all influence the outcome of the referral. Transitional stages are a time when the relationships between user and faceworkers are of special importance. Changes may be disturbing and the users may need time and help to get used to new faces and places. It may be most important to them when moving into residential care to have continuity of support provided by familiar faceworkers, whilst adjusting to the new situation and whilst a *handover* process is taking place. As well as *handing-on*, the process of *handing-back* may also require transitional work; for instance, in the case of a user who, during a period of intensive help, has had a close relationship with a primary faceworker which has to be terminated by a return to a previous faceworker.

When a user is receiving *concurrent help* from more than one faceworker, the form of working relationship may be parallel, interlocking or interactive or conjoint. Work runs in *parallel* when two or more methods of help are provided simultaneously, without any need for co-ordination of methods or contact between helpers. Indeed, there may be a positive need for them not to be in contact. For instance Mrs Hill the depressed single parent (Chapter 3) who was receiving counselling help from the social worker, might not have wished anyone in the self-help group to know about

74

this. *Interlocking work* is essential for carrying out different tasks within one method or for the integration of two help-methods when the input of workers needs to fit exactly with each other. In *conjoint work* the input of individual practitioners is closely confected within one method of help; for instance, where two workers are engaged in family or marital therapy. *Interactive work* is needed for tasks or methods which interweave in such a way that attitudes and feelings are inevitably involved. This is the area of complex collaboration. In the case of Len Leigh, the landscape gardener (Chapter 6), a development took place from parallel to interactive work.

In the structure of group discussions, I distinguish between *case meetings*, which are composed of faceworkers in the absence of the user, and *participatory meetings*, in which the user is present. In case meetings the primary purpose is objectivity in addressing the situation, applying professional knowledge and experience, at the same time expressing relevant subjective feelings in order that they may add to the ultimate objectivity of the deliberations. In communicating factual information and specific opinion, precision and brevity are of value, but the discussion of relevant feelings usually takes longer. In a participatory meeting users are no longer cases but people. The style of communication is different since its primary purpose is to engage the participation of user and/or carer in the group process, in order to fulfil the meeting's purpose. Mrs Newman, the would-be adopter (Chapter 6) is an example of the communication of feeling in a case meeting, and the example of Oliver Ogden, the aggressive adolescent (Chapter 6) explores the communication of feeling in a participatory meeting. *Conferences*, whether case or participatory, are similar but larger and usually more formal.

The confederate structure

Helper-groups are task groups set up for secondary and/or participatory collaboration. They are often composed of a *core-group* and an *extended group* and may take the form of a self-help group or a group of workers. The latter may be permanent, organised to provide certain methods of help to a succession of users; or they may be *specific*, set up on a once-off basis to meet a particular user's situation. Permanent groups, for example a team or a setting group, such as a ward or residential unit, have an *operational authority structure*, linked to, but sometimes distinct from , the professional and managerial accountability structure of line management. Even if decisions are taken by consensus, ultimate responsibility and decision-making power is known to reside in the hands of the *operational leader*, to whom it has been allocated by agreement between agency and/or professional managers. When managerially defined structures are not available, workers have to rely on a confederate structure. This is usually the case when collaboration crosses agency boundaries, even though for certain categories of trouble clear procedures and guidelines have been promulgated.

A *confederacy* is 'a union by league or contract between persons, bodies of men, or states, for mutual support or joint action; an alliance, a compact'. I see helpers, including the self-helper, as colleagues within a confederacy, forming an alliance for mutual support and a help-compact for joint action in dealing with a particular situation. The essential feature of the *confederate group* is that its members collaborate by volition. No worker has control over another from a different agency unless this has been agreed at managerial level. A confederacy is an operational structure with no built-in operational authority.

Practitioners are accountable to, and subject to the control of, their professional ethic and, with the exception of some medical practitioners, to a managerial senior of their own profession within their agency. In taking decisions which affect the group as a whole, unless one of the practitioners has statutory authority in the case, the views of all members are nominally of equal validity. *Influential power* comes from the relative importance of the input of the various workers and their agencies, from the practitioner's professional and personal standing and the faceworkers' ability to present their points-of-view. Self-helpers and carers may hand over their power to practitioners, but this can only be required of them when the latter have *statutory authority.*

A confederate structure is usually set up for a specific help-compact but in many settings which provide interprofessional care, there is a general confederate group of practitioners who work closely together for a good deal of their time. There are three main types of confederacy: link-up, core-group and network. For co-operation or simple collaboration all that may be necessary is a confederate *link-up*, which establishes lines of communication. Very often a few telephone calls or one meeting is sufficient for workers to achieve an integrated help-compact. It is not so much a question of how often or for how long workers meet, as the kinds of relationship that are formed and processes that take place when they do. For complex collaboration a *confederate core-group* is needed, in which helpers can confer together and relational interaction takes place. In the case of Melvin Manson (Chapter 6), the workers had only established a link-up; this was inadequate to their collaborative task. If a core-group had been established, its constitution would have had to be considered, using the principle of MEC. For instance, whether both the unit head and the worker allocated specially to Melvin should have been included; also whether Melvin himself, as a self-helper, and his mother, as an important carer and concurrent user should be there. The constitution of the core-group usually affects the shape and development of the help-compact. The selection of relevant helpers will depend partly on the helping approach of the worker setting up the group, partly on practical considerations, such as finding a time when everyone can meet, and on time priorities. If relevant people are not included, then adequate communication with them needs to be established. In complex cases, separate discussions cannot replace the interactional process of a group meeting; nor can trust be so easily established between people who never meet face-to-face. This is clearly illustrated by the meeting concerned with Mrs Newman, and the placement of Pam (Chapter 6).

The task of establishing a core-group is undertaken by the worker who both sees the need for it and feels sufficiently responsible for the case to expend the time. 'Whose meeting?' (Chapter 6) illustrated the point. By and large, if it is thought that a confederate group might be useful, the sooner it is established the better. So often when the helping process is going badly and workers finally get together, someone will voice the common thought: 'If only we had met before'.

In the country and small towns, practitioners and other helpers often know each other well and have formed good working relationships. In densely populated areas, because of overlapping administrative boundaries, the number of practitioners, their rapid turnover and the volume, complexity and urgency of problems, this is not so easy. Here the combination of faceworkers frequently varies from case to case, and new working relationships have to be made rapidly.

If workers are already involved in a case the first task on meeting is to describe their current responsibilities, help-methods and relationship with the user, in order to construct out of the separate help-compacts, an overall help-compact. This process can also serve to develop mutual understanding and trust and consolidate a working alliance. The help-compact finally agreed needs to be based either on positive consensus or else on an openly accepted compromise. For MEC, the number of meetings must be kept to a minimum. Thus in a first meeting it is essential to establish a structure for co-ordination and continuing communication and to agree the allocation of special roles.

Special facework roles

A *role* is a particular part to be played by an individual or group, in relation to another individual or group, or in fulfilling a task. Where there is complex collaboration there are probably at least two special roles to be filled; these are the function-roles of *primary faceworker* and *care co-ordinator*. Because they may be combined they have often become confused in the term key worker.

When the situation around Melvin Manson (Chapter 6) was looked at in the discussion group, it became obvious why each worker had assumed the position of the key worker. The probation officer had a specific authority, mandated by a court of law, which could not be delegated, and he had been seeing Melvin regularly. The GP had had a long and important contact with him, and this was likely to continue after the other workers' help would have ended. The residential worker was in the closest relationship with the user at the particular time. Each had interpreted the term 'key worker' in a way which justified their claim to it. Each had an important role, but these were not the same.

The role of *care co-ordinator* in this case was split into two sub-roles: *health co-ordinator*, carried continuously by the GP, and *social co-ordinator*, carried at the time of the discussion by the probation officer. This would end with the ending of the probation order but, if he thought Melvin still needed social care and with the latter's agreement, he might pass this role on to an area or voluntary agency social worker. Because of this division of responsibilities between health and social care, there may be a need to allocate specifically the further role of *general care co-ordinator*. At this particular time in the help-compact it would seem to belong to the probation officer because he had a mandatory responsibility in the case, and it was he who had initiated the residential placement.

The role of care co-ordinator carries responsibility for ensuring that services are co-ordinated, methods integrated and the help-compact reshaped to meet changing needs. Where collaboration crosses agency boundaries and is not therefore supported by agency structures, this role is of particular importance. Its function is to co-ordinate rather than to manage, because the relationships of those involved are of a confederate rather than bureaucratic nature. The role of care co-ordinator gives a worker no authority to enforce, but only to urge, that workers should co-operate and, where necessary, collaborate. In practice, if such collaboration is to be effective, it must always be based on volition or else it will be subtly undermined, as the nursery head in the case of Mrs Anson, the day nursery mother (Chapter 2) was well aware. If an agency has statutory authority for the management of certain types of case, the formal role of *care manager* may be designated, and this will inevitably include the functions of a general care co-ordinator.

In straightforward situations the user or a relative may co-ordinate their own help, although a health co-ordinator is generally potentially present in that virtually everyone has a GP. A social co-ordinator is only necessary if social help is complex or long-term. The more complex the helping-task, particularly if social and health care are both involved, the more likely that co-ordination will need to be undertaken by a practitioner. Whether the role of general care co-ordinator should be carried by a faceworker from health care or social care depends on the predominant nature of the trouble and respective responsibilities of the agencies. Who the actual worker should be depends on the likely degree of involvement of any particular service, and the relevant skills of particular workers. On the health side, it might be a health visitor, a district or hospital nurse, CPN, GP or medical consultant; on the social side, a faceworker from a number of different statutory or voluntary agencies, and from in- out- or day care settings.

The role of *primary faceworker* is carried by the helper with whom the user has the most important interface contact at any particular time. If the help-compact includes a relational method, such as counselling or therapeutic work, the worker carrying it out is likely to be the primary faceworker.

For Melvin Manson, at the time of the discussion, this was the residential worker. When the time came for him to leave the unit he might need another worker to fulfil the role of primary faceworker. It might revert to the probation officer, who held it earlier, or the GP who held it earlier still and who, in the future, might fulfil it on a regular or a periodic basis. Thus the carrier of the role may change as the help-compact changes. Here the process of handover is important, so that the user's natural disturbance at change and distress at loss does not create ill-feeling towards the new situation or worker. The role of primary faceworker may be combined with that of co-ordinator. Before Melvin went into the residential unit the two roles would have been carried by the probation officer; before that, by the GP.

There are many permutations in the roles of care co-ordinator and primary faceworker. Where collaboration is straightforward roles are assumed naturally and do not need to be made explicit. It is, as always, in complex situations that there is need for clarification, particularly when several practitioners have important input into the case, and more particularly when they share the same skills. A group structure in which roles and tasks are allocated serves an important function in containing and defusing rivalries. In the case of Melvin, when the three practitioners could see the importance they each had in fulfilling their role as part of a confederate group rather than in isolation, they were able to replace a rivalrous relationship with a working alliance.

When the help-compact includes various types of help in different settings, there may be concurrently more than one primary faceworker, covering well-differentiated spheres of help. For instance if a user with learning difficulties is living at home and going to a day centre, they may be getting special help there from a particular worker, in the role of primary worker, whilst at home the mother is probably the primary carer helped by the father and a number of friends and neighbours. She may also be the *informal care co-ordinator*, collaborating with a practitioner who co-ordinates the formal care and carries the role of general co-ordinator.

Networks

Full use of the potential resources is achieved through adequate knowledge, user-friendly referral systems, and the building of *helping networks*.

Network is a term used in so many different ways that in any particular context its use must be defined. The essence of a network is the interlinking of elements to make a loosely connected whole. It often contains a *nucleus* and an *extended* section. A structured network has well-established connections; an unstructured one, informal links only. *Helper-networks* are made up of people and are either specific or general. A *specific network* is set up to meet the needs of a particular user. *General networks* form part of the collaborative infrastructure which facilitates the building of specific networks.

Resource networks are made up of services for comprehensive and co-ordinated provision in a particular field of help, and depend on planning at managerial level. However, the actual use of a resource network depends to a large extent on the faceworkers and whether they know what is available and how to access it.

This can be facilitated by general *worker-networks* which have some permanency and which can have different focal points. The focus may be: a particular locality and/or particular field of help – for example a worker-network concerned with mental health in a local area and the services available to its residents; an agency, with its own network of working contacts relevant to the agency's functions; or a particular practitioner with a network of contacts useful to their work. There is a strong tendency for practitioners to see themselves or their agency at the centre of every network. At a meeting when participants were asked to draw a diagram of the network of services relevant to mental illness in their area, all drew either a diagram which had their agency or themselves at the centre. None put the local population, i.e. the potential users of the services at the centre of the network.

Agency-centred networks, often structured as *agency liaison groups*, and *practitioner-centred networks* are both of great value but, because they are centred on one part of the whole resource network, they tend towards a restricted viewing-point, with a bias towards their own input, rather than seeing themselves as one part of a comprehensive service for a particular set of users.

A group for mental health

The residential therapeutic community mentioned in the case of Melvin Manson, held regular meetings of its agency liaison group. Workers who came from other agencies concerned with mental health in the locality found this valuable but felt that the group should not be orientated solely to the unit, but to all relevant agencies. After some discussion, it was agreed that this group should be reconstituted as a group for mental health in part of the borough, and all agencies would have an equal place; there would in fact be no central agency and the group would be run by a committee. The group's boundary would no longer be that of the catchment area of a particular agency but the boundary of the local area.

The setting up of this group is described in a later chapter. I mention it here in order to illustrate the shift in viewing-point which is required in the move from an agency-centred to a *locality-centred* or *local network group*. It led to a widening of perspectives and a more comprehensive view of the available resources; participants learnt more about the functions of other workers and their agencies, with greater understanding of their strengths and their constraints. However because it was not agency-based it lacked a secure foundation and adequate sponsorship, despite the strong commitment of many of its members.

Whatever form worker networks take they contribute to an infrastructure which helps faceworkers to construct a user's specific network. In addition to those within the helping services, there are many *ordinary-life networks* from which help for a particular user can be drawn. These include the *personal networks* of extended family, friends, neighbours and workmates; then *local community networks*, which are based on a wide variety of common concerns, for example race, religion, educational and leisure activities, tenants' associations. If a community approach is to be promoted, certain workers in the formal services need a full knowledge of community resources and close working contacts with key people in the neighbourhood.

The construction of a specific network may be carried out by the particular user, an informal or formal carer, or it may be a joint undertaking. Often members of a family mobilise themselves into a core-group, to carry responsibility for planning and providing help for one of its number, and drawing on ordinary life networks. Such networks often operate as an undeclared part of the personal helping services, without any intervention from the formal carers, particularly when troubles are psychological or social, less so with problems of physical or serious mental ill-health. Formal carers are called in when the need is recognised for their knowledge, skills or access to resources.

For many help-compacts for home care, the user as self-helper, the carer and one or two of the formal carers are likely to form both a confederate core-group and the nucleus of a helping network. They serve different purposes. That of the core-group is to plan, make decisions and implement the help-compact; of the nuclear group, to create around itself a specific network to contribute to the help-compact. Its task is to find and enlist helpers who have the necessary human and material resources – for instance neighbours or those who offer respite care; to define their tasks and responsibilities; integrate them into the help-compact in the right relationship to the user and each other; establish lines of communication; and enable helpers to fulfil their part in the network, to their own and the core group's satisfaction. This is the process of *network-building* or *networking*.

Interconnection of the various types of helper group

By way of illustration I give the following example from a paediatric setting. It shows how in a single case a setting group, team, core-group, and networks of formal and informal carers were all needed and how they were co-ordinated.

Co-ordination of care

In a paediatric ward of an inner-city district hospital, the consultant had fostered a highly developed pattern of collaborative care for long-term cases. These were children with severe illnesses who required regular out-patient appointments and periodic hospitalisation. This meant that close integration was needed between in- and out- care. In some cases the consultant liked to call a case conference of as many of the workers as possible, but even if no conference were called smaller meetings were often arranged. His purpose was to help faceworkers appreciate that their input was part of a whole and, through discussion, to integrate and develop the care-compact.

Within the hospital there were regular ward meetings – the setting-group – at which the child would be discussed. In addition the consultant might occasionally hold a team meeting of those who were working closely together to help the particular child while in hospital. This team would probably include a registrar, houseman, sister, nurse, social worker and perhaps the teacher, play therapist, physiotherapist, occupational therapist. Hospital workers would all be subject to the operational authority of the consultant, who liked his decision to emerge as the result of group discussion. Confection of team members' tasks would be achieved through team discussion, based on already defined responsibilities and structures. The consultant also headed a confederate core-group, in which he had no operational authority although much influence, deriving from the authority of his position. This group included the parents and social worker, the ward sister and perhaps others who were particularly involved in the case. The group's composition matched its function: that of carrying the major responsibilities for overall planning and decision-making.

When the child was living at home, a different set of workers was involved, including some of the following: GP, district nurse, health visitor, headteacher, class and remedial teacher, home tutor, school doctor, educational psychologist, educational welfare officer, Invalid Children's Aid, NSPCC or other voluntary sector worker. There would be no pre-existing structures to co-ordinate the tasks of these individual workers with the hospital. It was a specific part of the paediatric social worker's job to carry the role of social and general co-ordinator. Through creating an agency network she had facilitated this role which had two aspects: co-ordinating the out-care services and maintaining links between out-care and in-care workers. Specific health care co-ordination was ensured through collaboration between the hospital medical staff, GP and school doctor. The fact that the care-compact was hospital-orientated made it easy to designate co-ordinating roles.

The description given by the hospital social worker of her contacts following a case-conference made it clear that unless such a co-ordinating role had been part of her task some of the value of the conference would have been lost through lack of continuing communication and feedback between the participants. From time to time she needed to talk on the phone or arrange a small meeting with a few of those who needed to confer together.

The parents were the nucleus of an informal network, composed of relatives, friends and neighbours. These helped in various ways so that the parents could give adequate time to their other children. The paediatric social worker had found that personal carers often built up their own informal network, but sometimes they needed help from the practitioner. Then she and the carer or carers involved would together form the network nucleus.

To build specific networks easily and quickly each agency and faceworker need to be clear what they require in terms of local knowledge, individual and network contacts. They need to avoid wasting time on contacts that are not essential for fulfilling their functional role. Very often one key contact can provide knowledge concerning a whole area of help, particularly when linking in to the local community.

The resource pool

This is the sum total of the help available to a particular person or family living in a particular locality. When the helping-approach is user-centred and community orientated, rather than profession-centred and agency orientated, the resource pool takes on a different look. It is usually conceived in terms of the organisations providing help. In Figure 7.1, I show two other ways of viewing the resource pool which are often more relevant when constructing a help-compact. The diagrams can be applied to help in general or a particular field of help, a particular locality or a particular user. The model on which they are constructed places the users at the centre of the resource pool as potential self-helpers, contributing to their own help-compact. Surrounding them are the faceworkers, the human face of help-provision. In Figure 7.1(a), the resource pool is classified according to setting; in Figure 7.1(b), according to the main purpose of the particular source of help. Here, special-help agencies provide specialised help for a particular category of trouble or user; self-help groups are composed of users who share similar troubles. General-help agencies provide the kind of help that everybody may need at some time in their life. The ordinary-life sector includes personal networks, community organisations and the para-helping services.

A community care approach emphasises the importance of this last-mentioned sector and extends the range of potential helpers. The input of practitioners, though likely to become rather different, is unlikely to be less, and there will be a greater need for close collaboration. An integrative approach does not weaken the boundaries between agencies or different types of helper. In recognising their validity it emphasises the need to clarify the differences of input and the areas of overlap, in order to make full use of each potential source of help.

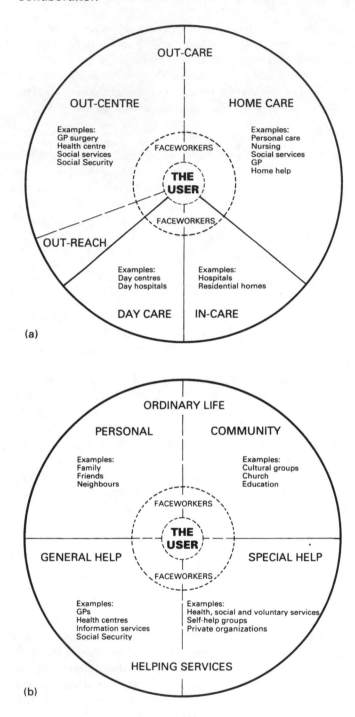

Fig. 7.1   The resource pool. (a) Settings of help and (b) main purposes served.

Chapter 8
Practitioners, Carers and Volunteers

The motivation of carers and volunteers has no element of financial gain: personal carers are often in need of care for themselves; local carers and volunteers may be in need of support; practitioners have professional skills, authority and accessing ability which puts them in a power-position. These are three important features in relationships between these sets of helpers.

Fulfilment of the principle of maximum self-responsibility for the user will be facilitated if the principle of maximum devolution down the line is adopted by those with the power to allocate tasks and responsibilities. This means that practitioners ensure that carers and volunteers can, if they wish and with adequate support, teaching and monitoring, take on skilled tasks. Provided they are not exploited, the full use of their abilities is likely to increase their personal satisfaction. The process of modelling is relevant here. If the person in a power-position manifests a particular relational model, the one in a less powerful position may well incorporate the model and use it in a similar situation. Giving maximum responsibility down the line is a likely way of ensuring that the user at the end of the line also has maximum self-responsibility.

In home care, besides their specific functions, practitioners have a large shared domain, which includes network-building and relational work. Once a specific network has been established, its maintenance may need input from a practitioner to support both the personal and local carers, sorting out difficulties and actively appreciating their contribution.

It is well known that carers carry a heavy load, both physically and emotionally. If they do not have family and friends who are able to relieve their stress, the practitioner should view the carer as a potential concurrent user. Through relational work with the user and carer separately or together, feelings which are inevitably mixed and often include guilt, can be aired and accepted, increasing mutual understanding and togetherness. Through the help of a third party, members of a family can find a balance between egoism and altruism, ensuring that every member of the family, not only the user, has as good a quality of life as possible.

Self-help groups

The importance of empowerment to users and carers is demonstrated by the growth of the self-help movement and the development of self-help groups. They serve various purposes: mutual help, social activities, action on behalf of the members. In relation to such groups, practitioners are in a very different power-position from their usual relationship with the user. Groups may be totally independent of formal help or use it in various ways: practical back-up, such as room-space or finance; help in setting up and organising the group; or provision of professional services integrated into the group's programme. The practitioner has a complex relationship with the members of these groups, the balance of power, through shared responsibility, being of paramount importance to the latter. The more that users and carers are empowered, the more is the practitioner's general responsibility of a reactive nature. Their proactive responsibility is then confined to the province of their special skills, which may well be of great help to those in the group, if proffered within a collaborative relationship.

In many group situations, as the helping process develops, the balance of responsibility shifts. The following example shows how practitioners gradually reduced their proactive responsibility and eventually drew out from a situation in which carers felt empowered to take over.

Rehabilitation and a self-help group

In a district hospital, people who were about to return home with some disability were offered a number of sessions in a group run by a social worker, an occupational therapist and a speech therapist, all of whom they already knew. This group gave its members the opportunity to discuss their problems with others in a similar situation. Those with a speech disability found it particularly helpful to hear someone else voice the feelings they experienced but could not easily express. They all had emotional as well as practical problems about living at home again. Some of them also used the group to share feelings of distress, depression, anger and frustration. The aim of the workers in the group was to further rehabilitation and to help in the transitional stage between hospital and home care. Users who had just gone home could still come to the group. The confection of relational help with practical advice was of particular importance, this input being provided by the social worker and the occupational therapist respectively.

On one occasion, a man questioned whether he would be able to get on and off a bus. He did not seem satisfied with the suggestions that were offered for enlisting help, and finally said: 'I shall feel a right Charlie, if I have to get someone to help me. After all I'm not that old'. This feeling of embarrassment was shared by others, some saying they would rather not try to travel on a bus, but others said they would make sure that people took notice of them. The practitioners encouraged the group both to discuss their feelings about having a handicap and to look for practical ways of minimising its effects.

In the course of running these groups, different staff took part, and at one stage the hospital social worker was replaced by an area social worker, who wished to work closely with the hospital at the transitional stage for these users. This transboundary process led to a cross-fertilisation of ideas, which brought about a further project. In a hall in the locality, a monthly group for those now living at home was started by three of the practitioners. Both users and carers came to it. It served as social and lunch club, and a place where the practitioners could function in an informal way. Sometimes there were discussions about practical and emotional problems in the same way that there had been in the hospital group, but now the carers also participated.

After a time, the question arose as to whether this project was duplicating the work of the local day centre and the hospital and whether it was a good use of practitioner time. It was the personal carers who were determined to keep the project going, because they were getting something from it which they did not get elsewhere. They began to take over responsibility for the group, and this enabled the practitioners to minimise their input.

There can be difficulties on both sides in sharing responsibility. Practitioners may fear that if they draw back too far the user will not be getting the best help. They may feel anxious that they are not doing their job properly. Members of self-help groups may feel that to be dependent on practitioners puts them in their power or, at least, in an inferior position. They may therefore reject help which could be of value or, in accepting it, fear or resent the worker who provides it. In the above example, it was the practitioners who started the group, involved the carers and worked with them in a changing balance of responsibility. Sometimes it is the other way round, a self-help group enlisting the services of a practitioner; then initiative and the power to allocate tasks is in the hands of the self-helpers rather than the practitioner.

In either situation it is necessary for practitioners to define for themselves the nature and extent of their special professional skills and powers and to be able to discuss their contribution with group members. If user and carer empowerment is a valued principle, practitioners must consider their assumptions about norms and their judgements about the relative merits of one or another lifestyle, self-monitoring the use of their professional power of influence. An open attitude and flexibility are needed if a working alliance is to be established.

Practitioners and volunteers

Usually it is the volunteer who is employed to support or extend the work of the practitioner and then the volunteer is incorporated into the organisational structure. In the following example the opposite is the case: a practitioner is introduced into a project run by a group of volunteers in order to extend its work.

Patrick Potter: problem volunteer

An old terrace house was used for a centre with the dual purpose of making money for the local association of MIND and offering a place in which those with mental health troubles could become involved in useful or leisure activities, in a friendly atmosphere. The centre comprised a shop selling good second-hand clothes, bric-à-brac and new things; a sewing-room for repairing or making things; a coffee-bar with a large sitting area where befriending and counselling went on in an informal way, a room in which groups and classes could be held; a small room for individual counselling, as well as offices, storerooms and a small garden. Lunch clubs, day and evening social clubs were held on the premises. The project was staffed by volunteers, a shop-manager receiving an honorarium and, after a time, by one paid professional worker – an occupational therapist with experience in the mental health field. A few of the key volunteers, including those who had conceived and set up the project, formed a management committee, which was accountable to the local association's executive committee.

The people who came into the centre might be customers in the shop or coffee-bar, a member of a club or class, or a volunteer working in the shop, coffee-bar or workroom. Those who had mental health troubles were never differentiated or identified as users of help. When allocating work, the committee had to assess new volunteers according to their competence and degree of vulnerability.

The professional's skills were used to extend the methods of help and widen the range of people who might benefit from them. She provided skilled help for those with mental health troubles who used the centre, and for supporting and increasing the skills of the key volunteers. She increased the centre's contacts with various local hospitals and social work agencies, thus facilitating referrals either for membership of clubs and classes or for work as a volunteer. Making contact with the formal agencies was the professional worker's exclusive domain, but other of her functions were shared by some of the volunteers who, though without formal training, had considerable skill in using individual and group relational methods. Such facework methods were used in the context of the setting methods, which were based on the provision of a friendly and tolerant atmosphere in which groups of people either worked together to make money for MIND or enjoyed a leisure activity together.

Because there were a great many vulnerable volunteers, the committee decided that, apart from those in key positions, volunteers should only work in the centre for four half-days a week. This rule was explained to newcomers and, although some wanted to come more often, they accepted the rule. Patrick Potter was the exception; he insisted on coming even when not on the rota. When asked not to do this, he became aggressive and threatening. At first the committee gave in to him, but then they decided that the rule-breaking must stop. They planned that the next time it happened the practitioner should be called to see if she could persuade him to conform. She got Patrick to sit down with her on their own. They discussed the question of accepting rules and having to share with others. She also expressed her understanding of the painfulness of being deprived of what was of value to him. They continued to have an occasional talk together and Patrick settled down, although still now and again trying to break the rule.

The value of a controlling relationship within a friendly atmosphere is apparent. As a result, Patrick began to gain greater self-control when his wishes were thwarted. The key volunteers also learned that limit-setting was a benevolent function. Facing the problem of threatening behaviour in this particular situation led to contact being made with the local community policeman and a procedure was clarified should police help be needed. Another resource was enlisted which enabled the centre to help a wider range of people.

This situation illustrates how developments can grow from the collaboration of practitioner and volunteers. At the beginning considerable effort had to be made to enable the relationship to develop creatively. The process the workers went through to achieve this demonstrates certain collaborative difficulties which are likely to occur at the interface between practitioner and volunteer.

Practitioner and volunteer

The idea of employing a paid professional at the centre described above came from the director of the local association. The executive committee of the organisation approved the idea and funds were raised. Although members of the centre committee appeared to fall in with the plan, it turned out later that they had not backed it wholeheartedly and had not openly discussed their mixed feelings. Some months after the professional worker – Mary – had started, it became clear that things were not going well. She could not find her proper role and the volunteers were dissatisfied.

I was asked to help sort out the problem and attended meetings with the centre committee, Mary and the director. Gradually much hostility began to be expressed, because the decision to employ a practitioner had been taken by the executive committee without full consultation with the centre committee, the members of which were covertly affronted and angry. These feelings, which had nothing to do with the practitioner herself, had increased their hostility towards her and they had to be worked through before looking at the specific difficulties of incorporating a paid practitioner.

Here one of the common causes of collaborative failure is operating, already identified in the case of Daisy, the paediatric patient (Chapter 2): background tensions which do not originate in the particular working relationship but are influencing it negatively.

A similar difficulty had to be worked through concerning the introduction of a group consultant to the centre committee. Again the committee felt that this had been effected after insufficient discussion, nor did they fully understand my function. Hostility was manifest in subtly polite terms but eventually the group began to see the value of expressing their views more directly. They found that I was not upset by their negative response and the discussion led to a better understanding. Then it became possible to look at their problems with the practitioner.

Before she had arrived, key volunteers were unconcerned with job descriptions and formalised accountability. They worked together as a group of friends, who only needed to organise themselves and define their tasks sufficiently to carry through what they had set out to do. The centre's style allowed for a great deal of personal initiative, which could sometimes get out of hand but which helped to maintain a lively and creative ethos. There were the normal ups and downs in a group which had considerable cohesion and confidence.

At first, committee members began hinting that Mary did not seem to do anything and made no difference to the centre; that she had no useful answers when they asked her advice about difficult volunteers. A few meetings later they began to express feelings that things had not gone so well since Mary's advent, though they did not know why. Somehow the atmosphere was different and they did not enjoy their work so much. Mary was full of praise for the way in which they coped with disturbed people and incorporated them into the work of the centre. Then a volunteer said: 'But I feel you know what you are doing, while we just rely on our feelings and common sense'. Mary: 'That is what is so good about the way you help. You are so spontaneous and friendly'. The reply: 'But now you are here, we realise how little we know about mental illness and the right way to help'.

Much more was said along these lines, and it became clear that the presence of a trained worker had presented a great threat to the volunteers, causing them to doubt their own ability. At first they had coped with this by belittling Mary's usefulness. Once she had found her feet, her contribution to the work of the centre could not be denied. Envy and rivalry must inevitably have been present, although they were never openly expressed. The volunteers seemed to be dealing with such feelings through denial of their own competence, rather than Mary's. The positions were now reversed, and it was Mary who could do everything and they who were not much use. The more she reassured them, the more they felt her superiority.

It emerged that from time to time in the past they had experienced insecurity in running the centre, but this had greatly increased when they felt that a professional eye was being cast over their work. They felt at a disadvantage because of Mary's qualifications though, at the same time, they felt in an advantageous position because of their age and life experience relative to hers. The various differences between them were an inevitable cause of comparison which spoiled the previous pleasant atmosphere. Realising the benefit that Mary brought to the centre, they found the situation even more difficult to manage, and felt unhappy and angry.

In most relationships between practitioners and volunteers, the practitioner is in the more powerful position, but in this case, the key volunteers were both in the majority and, as committee members, in charge of running the centre. However, despite this, they seemed to feel impotent, unable to do anything to change the situation. They reiterated that they felt they were not much good. It appeared to be Mary's presence which had deskilled them rather than any particular thing that she had said or done. In fact, she was an unassuming person who would not normally upset people or constitute a threat. There was a strong polarisation on the parameter of competence, which eventually was verbalised. At this point Mary said: 'I feel I must share with you that I have felt extremely anxious here. More so than in any other job I've had. The way you cope makes me question what my qualification is worth. Is it just a piece of paper?' The uncertainty-in-role which had been experienced by the volunteers was also felt by the professional. The deskilling effect of their working side-by-side was mutual. Once this was out in the open, it became possible to recognise their different contributions and acknowledge the value of one without having to diminish the value of the other. In the ensuing meetings, a process of clarification followed, looking realistically at skills, responsibilities, motivation and commitment, and discussing how the differences they had identified could complement each other.

It was recognised that the relational skills of the key volunteers were enhanced by their concern, friendliness and life experience and through sharing tasks with the others. The difference between the strong and the vulnerable volunteers was real but not divisive. As a result the ex-patient could identify with the group; a volunteer amongst volunteers, doing something useful and 'belonging'. Although the practitioner could be equally caring, the nature of the relationship with the vulnerable volunteer was inevitably different because of her professional role. Collaboration over time brought positive developments: Mary became more spontaneous and flexible in her working relationships, and the key volunteers understood more about the nature of psychological difficulties and how to help people.

Certain tensions remained. The differentiating boundary between paid and unpaid worker, occasionally caused problems. Although key volunteers had their allotted hours, they very often worked longer when something needed to be done. There was an expectation that the paid worker would do the same, in fact that, being paid, she should be even readier to do so. Mary felt that she had contracted for a given number of hours and although she sometimes volunteered to work on, she should not be made to feel guilty if she did not. This difference was never resolved but was tolerated. It had a rational basis which could be easily grasped and, although causing irritation, it did not undermine confidence.

We see here how background tensions had compounded the inevitable difficulties of complex role-relationships. The complexity arose from a lone professional working alongside unqualified volunteers who at the same time were members of the committee responsible for running the project. Uncertainty-in-role was inevitable. Whether or not Mary had unwittingly coped with her initial insecurity by using her professionalism to deskill the volunteers and so make herself feel superior, her very presence had been enough to do so. Once the uncertainty-in-role could be talked about, relationships began to change. Acceptance of differences led to mutual respect and positive interaction. Practitioners may sometimes feel unsure of their skills when working alongside other qualified workers, but volunteers who have considerable capacity seem to pose an equal, if not stronger, threat.

Volunteers are often well suited to facework and able to carry out some of the tasks of a practitioner. In times of unemployment or cuts, the introduction of volunteers into the statutory services may be feared as a way of replacing paid workers. However, work roles for volunteers can usually be defined in such a way as to meet the fear of job losses. A greater hindrance to their involvement is likely to be the uncertainty-in-role raised in the professional worker by competence in those without qualification, even when their position is by definition inferior.

The threat of volunteers

In the rehabilitation group described earlier, there came a time when hospital transport was difficult and members of the group who were to be picked up from home failed to come or else arrived very late. In my role as group consultant, I suggested that they might approach the Volunteers Bureau to see if escorts with suitable cars could be found, adding that the volunteers might also be useful in the group, by making tea and helping members to the toilet. The idea appeared to be well received but weeks went by and no action was taken. Good reasons were produced but finally I felt these must be rationalisations serving to cover some deeper reason. When I pressed the point, one practitioner said: 'They might pull the rug from under our feet'.

This practitioner was speaking for the whole group and shows their insecurity when working alongside volunteers. Self-evaluation by reference to others is a normal human process, and when there are clear divisions between people based on their role, qualifications and special skills, the issue of relative status is almost inevitable. It can easily lead to rivalry, as in the case of Melvin Manson (Chapter 6), or to uncertainty-in-role as in the examples given above. Recognition of such reactions is the first step to minimising their effect.

Hindrances to collaboration between the user and faceworker and between faceworkers themselves

In the foregoing chapters I have illustrated and discussed a range of relational problems which hinder collaboration. The root causes of these hindrances fall into four main categories: inadequate understanding of the subtle nature of helping relationships; a helping approach which is inadequate to the complex needs of users; a separatist attitude to helping; and maladaptive methods for coping with role-insecurity. The first root cause has been covered in Part 1, the last three will be discussed more fully in Part II.

Part II
Identity and Boundaries

Chapter 9
The Importance of Identity and Role

In trying to understand the hindrances to collaboration, I have found the concepts of identity, role and boundaries to be of great value. They throw light on the needs behind those separatist attitudes and defensive processes which hinder collaboration, and also on the empowerment of users. The basic human need for a *secure and satisfying identity* is identical for user and helper. For users, it underlies all their specific needs. For helpers, it is a root cause of the great value they often attach to their working role, since roles contribute to identity. In this chapter I give examples to show the importance of identity to users, carers and workers, in particular, practitioners, and discuss more fully the concepts of identity and role.

Role evaluation

The pecking order

During a lunch group for workers concerned with the under-fives in an inner-city locality, discussion turned on the relative status of the people involved with young children. Criteria by which this was determined gradually emerged, as agreement was reached on the following order: doctor, nursery matron, social worker, health visitor, nursery class teacher, nursery nurse, pre-school playgroup organiser and volunteer. There was one or more representative of each in the group. Everybody was in agreement about the top and the bottom of the order but there was considerable discussion about the middle. Authority was the factor on which the final decision rested: that of social workers, deriving from their statutory authority; of health visitors from their knowledge of child-rearing and their influence through advice-giving; of nursery class teachers, deriving from the intellectual standing of their profession and agency.

Towards the end of the discussion, a playgroup leader said: 'As an unpaid, untrained worker I come last, and as a mother I feel right at the bottom of the pile'.

Mothers are the carers who carry the greatest responsibility for the under-fives. This mother was highly skilled and confident in her mothering role and was responsible for a playgroup in which she helped others care for their children. Was the bottom of the pile the place where she should feel herself to be? If not, how had this come about? Partly I think because she had identified herself with the stereotype of the mothers who needed most help from the practitioners in the group. Partly because her self-image seems to have been reduced by comparison with people who had a professional role in relation to small children. Assessment of status was based on knowledge and skills which, for the mother, were general rather than specialised; and of authority, hers being personal, whilst the practitioners' was supplemented by the authority of profession and agency. The discussion about special skills, knowledge and authority must have influenced her self-evaluation although, as a generalist rather than a specialist in child care, she might have rated as highly as any of them. In another context, for instance the playgroup of which she had charge or her own home, she would have had a very different experience of her identity in the mothering role. Thus comparison is an important element in evaluating one's role. The values by which it is assessed may originate in the individual, a particular group, or society as a whole. In the above example, commonly held social values are operating as well as the values of professional workers.

The roles that people carry and the way they are evaluated by themselves and by others are vital to maintaining a good self-image. This affects how people feel about themselves which, in turn, can have a strong influence on how they function and relate to other people. This will influence how others perceive and relate to them, which in turn will influence how they feel about themselves. It is a subtle interactional process which can spiral in either direction.

The user's identity

A user is in a particular role, that of a person who has sought help, and in a *role relationship* with the person who can offer it. The *role-identity* of a user varies according to the type of relationship with the helper. This is determined by the agency, the helper and the user but, at the beginning of a helping process, the latter's influence is usually small.

The atmosphere of an agency may be formal or informal, impersonal or friendly. In setting the scene, this will affect users as they cross the threshold. Workers will be influenced in the way they relate to the user by the agency ethos and by their duties, training and personality. As a result, in their first contacts on entering an agency, users may have the experience of being defined in a certain way. They may find they have become a number, a body, important as an emergency or an interesting case, a social outcast, a failure, under suspicion of 'working the system'; or they may be of significance as a person with a trouble which needs help, with feelings and individuality, a potential collaborator. How users respond will depend on their state at the time and whether the defined *user-identity* fits their individual identity as well as on their habitual ways of refusing an unacceptable identity and contributing to its redefinition. Users with a forceful personality, or with an educational or financial status equal to the practitioner may assert their own identity, others may meekly or grudgingly conform or take a middle line.

Individual workers are in a strong position in determining role relationships. *Role-definition* should match the situation and is therefore closely related to the practitioner's input. If this changes during the helping process, the role relationship may need to change correspondingly. Being complementary, changes in one role inevitably require changes in the other. Since the process of role-definition often goes on at a low level of awareness it may be influenced by unrecognised needs; for instance that of users who enjoy being looked after and helpers who enjoy having others dependent on them.

The definition of a user-role is important in ensuring the triple aim of helping. Maximum self-responsibility and the users' rights to determine what constitutes optimum quality of life for themselves, require a participatory role. Personal integration and social integration require roles that integrate rather than fragment or ostracise. The triple aim of helping is, in fact, based on the need for a secure and satisfying identity.

Role-definition plays an important part in those help-methods that rely heavily on the setting, whether this be an old people's or a children's home, a ward or a therapeutic community. The MIND centre described in connection with Patrick Potter (Chapter 8) offers a good illustration of the relevance of role-definition to the helping process.

Redefining the role: the MIND centre

Everybody who crossed the threshold of the centre, with the exception of the one paid worker, was either a customer in the shop or coffee-bar, a volunteer selling, serving, sorting or making things to sell, or a member of a social or educational group. Some customers came just to shop, others dropped in frequently and might spend hours in the coffee-bar. There was no differentiation between those who did or did not have mental health troubles. It became evident that defining referred or potential users as volunteers, members or customers, was in itself a helpful process. It offered the opportunity to take on new roles which could influence a user's identity in a positive way.

Some who had been patients over a long period, although agreeing to become volunteers, resented the responsibilities, however minimal, which the role carried. They had become accustomed to having little expected of them or, if it were, that it would take the form of a passive response to the face-worker. They had developed an ineffectual identity, lacking a sense of personal value, purpose and responsibility, at the same time egocentric: in fact, 'a poor thing'. In the role of volunteer, they undertook some task, however simple, the primary purpose of which was not for their personal benefit but to make money for MIND. After a while, through carrying out a job in the centre, they became identified with their working group and its values: doing something useful for a good cause. They shared in the general pleasure when the week's takings were the highest ever.

The implicit boundary between 'strong' and 'vulnerable' volunteers, was recognised as defining responsibilities but did not devalue anybody. Through identifying with a friendly and purposive group, using and acquiring skills, the sense of identity with which a person with mental health problems had arrived was gradually modified. Many began to find greater meaning in their lives, with increased self-confidence and energy; a process of empowerment which showed in their relationships and activities. In the context of a kindly and boundary-setting system, some, such as Patrick Potter (Chapter 8), had the chance to work through a personal difficulty and develop a more mature response. The presence of the one practitioner did not disturb the basic pattern of role relationship between fellow volunteers or fellow members, but it made a practitioner-user relationship readily available should it be needed.

There is an imbalance of capability in any helping relationship, but this is often reinforced by role-definition. Even where practitioners guard against it, the user may try and push them into a superior position. This may be turned to good effect but all too easily the user's self-image is diminished and the practitioner's status invalidly enhanced, to the detriment of the identity of both. This was made clear in the health visitors' discussion (Chapter 5). All helpers are liable to operate this subtle form of 'user-abuse'. Conversely, enhancement of the user's self-image was demonstrated in the dialogue between the child psychiatrist and the parents (Chapter 5), where they were given a participatory role.

Within the sphere of the helping services, the roles of self-helper, mutual-helper, member, participant, volunteer, can be integrated with patient or client roles or run in parallel, as in the MIND centre. Whichever way is appropriate, the defining of *proactive roles* has a powerful effect in enabling people to cope with troubles.

The carer's identity

The carers are in a different position from workers in that their helping relationship is grounded in a personal relationship. Because of this their role is easily taken for granted and diminished by practitioners, whose professionalised role relationship ensures their status in the eyes of the world. When the user is ill or has a disability practitioners frequently treat carers as identical to workers, and overlook their possible need to be identified as concurrent users. Even if they do not need specific help, they need to be treated differently from a worker doing the same job; the user requires recognition as a person with their own identity and needs, not only as a person in role. Such recognition by a practitioner is a matter of attitude rather than time.

Empowerment of users and carers

It is usually practitioners who hold the power-position in defining roles. However users are seeking a more active part in this particularly over matters relating to natural processes such as birth and death. In both these situations greater *user-participation* is being demanded in the process of role-definition. If rightly used, role-definition clarifies the functions and responsibilities of the people concerned; wrongly used it can lead to an unjustified imbalance of power.

When people with a common interest form themselves into an identifiable group, individual identity is supplemented and strengthened by group identity. It takes time for the voice of a users' or carers' group to be sufficiently heard in the right quarters to bring about overall change. Meanwhile, through group identification and support, the enhanced identity of the individuals concerned is strengthened and begins to have its effect at ground level, influencing the practice of individual practitioners.

The practitioner's identity

Unlike users and carers the roles of practitioners are supported by their identification with profession and agency. These give them a strong role-identity, as the following conversation shows.

Out of uniform

> **A** social worker described how, walking down a hospital corridor, he met a lady who smiled at him. For a moment he did not recognise her. Then, realising she was a ward sister with whom he shared several cases, he stopped and said: 'For one moment I didn't recognise you out of uniform'. She replied: 'That doesn't surprise me. I feel quite different in my uniform. I'm a nurse, a sister. I'm somebody!' He replied: 'Somebody quite formidable!' They laughed.

The concept of identity

The concept of *identity* is a subtle one, having two apparently opposite meanings: first, that of sameness, sharing common qualities, being identical;

second, that of differentiation, having individuality. *Group identity* is the quality of uniqueness and cohesion which binds together people who are the same in some respect, the shared factor acting as a common denominator. This differentiates it from all other groups. *Individual identity* is the uniqueness and cohesion of a human being.

Identity has two aspects: *internal identity* is known subjectively, either inside the group or the individual; *external identity* is again known subjectively by members of the group or the individual but also by other people. In the latter case the *perceived identity* is coloured by the subjectivity of the viewer according to personality, values and preconceived ideas. The perceiver identifies a person or a group, names it and attaches pre-existing associations to it.

Human identity, whether in the form of a group or an individual, belongs to an organism existing for some purpose. This organism is a *system* with an internal organisation designed to sustain itself and carry out its functions, and an external boundary which separates it from its environment and other systems, across which intake, output and relationships take place. All living systems have potential for growth and change, stimulated by internal activity, external influences and feedback, the latter making possible self-evaluation and planning for change.

Individual identity has a core and an extended section. *Core-identity* is based on physical constitution, personal capacities, a *core personality* of emotional and relational patterns laid down early in life, and characteristics deriving from the culture of origin; it usually remains fairly constant throughout life. It is this which provides a continuing *sense of identity*, of being 'Me', 'Myself', to which the pronoun 'I' is ascribed. *Extended identity* develops as a result of maturation, the development of an *extended personality*, relationships, culture, education, acquisition of personal, social and working skills, new roles and group affiliations, and the effect of external events. From an early age, a protective *cover-identity*, mask or 'persona' is developed, hiding what is too personal to be exposed, and a *social identity*, through which to relate acceptably to others. The extended identity will vary at different stages of life – for instance, in youth or middle age – and according to the individual's emotional or material state, to identification with different groups and roles. In a similar manner groups have a core and extended identity, the first remaining constant, the latter subject to modification.

The human being is a system within systems and an individual's identity is always influenced by their psychological and social environment. If early upbringing and group influences have tended towards the development of an individualised and secure identity, a person can stand alone as an individual. If not, they rely for their sense of identity, to a greater or lesser degree, on the groups within which they are contained or the roles which they fulfil. To identify with some person, group or role means to become one with them. This can be a useful substitute for individual identity when a person's core identity is weak or unintegrated, and for everyone group-identification and role-identification are a support and an enhancer of their identity. The value of this for certain users was shown in the last example, Redefining the role: the MIND centre.

Internally experienced identity is linked to the *self-image*. This is a picture of themselves, subjectively experienced by individuals or groups, to which they ascribe values – good and bad, effective and ineffective, and so on. *Self-esteem* – the self-image evaluated – is an essential component of identity. It is measured against an *ideal self-image* to which the group or individual aspires but seldom reaches. Sometimes they identify with a good self-image, sometimes a bad one; most of the time, the self-image provides sufficient self-esteem and cohesion to support a stable sense of identity, good enough for getting along in life.

Most people have at some time experienced a *loss of identity* through change in circumstances, ending of a close relationship or loss of a role; an *identity crisis* may be experienced by a mother when her children leave home, or a man when he retires or is made redundant. When the experience of one's self as having value and one's life as having meaning is diminished, sense of identity suffers.

Roles

A *role* is a defined part to be fulfilled or carried by an individual or group, and there are several different types of role which are relevant to the helping relationship.

The *character role* is one which confers a descriptive title on the role-carrier and provides the bearer with a certain recognisable character, of, say, the user, carer, volunteer, practitioner. This *prototype role* is personalised and becomes an *individual role* when carried by a particular person.

The essential or *primary role characteristics* often have others added to them, so that the role is developed into a well-rounded figure, embodying attitudes, values and patterns of behaviour; but these secondary character-istics are modifiable. For instance the father role has certain basic char-acteristics such as provision and protection for the child, but the *secondary characteristics* of a present-day father have changed considerably from those of the Victorian father and provide a very different role-identity. Some professions have a well-defined role-identity, which provides a stereotype, a fixed image about which generalisations can be made. However profes-sional stereotyping is less easy that it used to be because, along with current changes in society, role characteristics are in a process of change.

Character roles are *composite roles* incorporating the *activity role*, based on the fulfilment of certain tasks; and the *relational role*, on certain patterns of relationship. For example there are certain activities normally carried out by a mother and certain patterns of relationship. Both these types of role contribute to the composite role of the mother. In any character role, one or other may predominate. In the character role of the practitioner activity roles and relational roles are closely confected.

A *function role* is based solely on the function to be carried out, such as that of a co-ordinator as discussed in Chapter 6.

A *complementary role* embodies a role relationship between two people or groups who carry *matching roles*; for instance mother and child, husband and wife, friends, helper and user, collaborators, agencies which together provide a comprehensive service.

Two other types of role are important to the helping relationship, which are personalised when enacted by people. The *modal role* embodies complementary patterns of manifestation; for example someone may fulfil an active, passive, dominant, submissive, authoritarian, responsible, dependent, loving or aggressive role in relation to another person. Modal roles may be manifested between strangers: the dominant/submissive role relationship may be observed between two people wanting to board a bus at rush hour. Within personal relationships, modal role relationships are always present. Although manifested, they are only ever known subjectively, and the way they are experienced and perceived internally and externally may be very different. A man in the paternal role may manifest it in a way which to the outside observer is perceived as a dominant manner, whilst he feels himself to be weak as a father, and may be experienced by his child as a tyrant. From examples given, it is clear that the modal role relationships in primary collaboration – particularly active/passive and responsible/dependent modes – are highly relevant to the identity of users and the help which they receive.

The *archetypal role* is the other relational role of importance in helping. It derives from an *archetypal image* – an embodied idea which seems fundamental and ever-present within humanity as a whole; the archetypal image of the father, mother, lover, child, priest, healer, benefactor, protector, guide, scapegoat, enemy, and many others. An archetypal image often brings with it charisma and the quality of being a little larger than life, and these may overshadow individual characteristics.

A complementary character role may be rooted in an archetypal role and then influenced by cultural and personal factors. Thus the complementary role of mother will contain archetypal relational patterns which seem to hold good throughout all humanity, supplemented by patterns belonging to a particular culture or mixture of cultures. This makes up the current prototype maternal role, which will then become individualised in the relational patterns belonging to a particular mother and her child. These will be influenced by the mother's personality and her own mothering experience as a child; by the particular child itself and the psychological and external circumstances surrounding its birth and early life. One mother may differ markedly from another but, though individual manifestations in the role are very diverse in content and relational quality, they are none the less always rooted in the archetypal role and influenced by the prototype role of a culture.

The same applies to the role of *the healer*. In ancient times and in primitive societies, man always seems to have needed the healer who has been identified with an archetypal image and invested with special knowledge, powers and authority. In modern society there still seems to be a need for the archetypal healer and a tendency to identify the doctor with this image; perhaps because people when ill wish to feel themselves in the hands of someone with exceptional powers. Nursing is also subject to identification with an archetypal image, that of the mother, with her functions of care and control at a physical level. When ill, people are often glad to hand over the responsibility of caring for themselves and revert to the position of a child. This archetypal mother image can be strengthened by being paired with the paternalistic role of the doctor. Social workers do not have an obvious underlying archetypal image, the profession having a number of different roots, and I think their authority derives more from statutory powers.

Role relationships and role identity

At any particular time people are never manifesting the whole of their identity. They are '*in role*' and have various *part-person identities* which fit their main character roles. These role-identities become attached to the core identity, and adopt the pronoun 'I'. In very close complementary roles, such as husband/wife, mother/child, much that is very personal will be manifest, and many acquired roles may be irrelevant for much of the time. In other role relationships, the personal may largely be irrelevant, although core personality is inevitably present in every relationship. People are probably unaware of being identified with only a part of themselves. For example the mother who also works as a practitioner will, while working, probably not be conscious of her mothering role, and vice versa, unless strong concerns draw her back to the other role.

People identify strongly with the roles which are important to them, and these will become an essential part of their self-image, and crucial to their sense of identity. It is this which gives roles their great significance, and may cause people in a power-position to shape relational roles in a way which supports their own identity. Role definition is a powerful process within primary collaboration. Modal role relationships in which power is unevenly distributed, can easily become incorporated into the character roles of practitioners and users. They may be taken for granted as core constituents when in fact they are extended elements which could be modified.

In the *self-helper role*, the interface between user and helper has been internalised. There is an inner role relationship between the two. Internal conversations may proceed in which the helper encourages the user to undertake tasks and behave sensibly, to take courage and keep on trying. The caring aspect of the helper is usually less evident in the internalised helping role, it is difficult for the internal helper to keep the comforting role untrammelled by self-pity. The drive for independence and equality of position are sometimes strong motivating forces in self-helpers, making it likely that people of this type can acknowledge their need to be cared for more easily in a self-help group than in a relationship with a practitioner. However, if definition of roles is undertaken within a collaborative relationship, it may be found that modal roles can be more evenly balanced and the relationship more acceptable to the user.

Participatory roles – those which require the user to take an active part – are common in day care and long-term residential settings. Here the role relationship is more likely to be with the institution or the group of workers, rather than a specific worker, evidenced by the user's identification as resident or member. Responsibilities and tasks on which participatory roles are based, when incorporated into the setting-method, are usually accepted without question. It is when there is a redefining of participatory roles that they are likely to be questioned by users and faceworkers alike because of the threat to their established identity.

In primary collaboration, users generally take a participatory role, but where they are engaged with more than one helper, as in participatory collaboration, the patterns of role relationship and the necessary skills for sustaining them are only now being developed. In a participatory group, the user's individual relationships to the various members of the group, will affect the relationships of the latter to each other. For example, Oliver Ogden, the aggressive teenager (Chapter 6), and his mother were empowered to participate actively and, as a result, the role relationships between the professionals were subtly changed from those pertaining during the case meeting held immediately before.

Identity and helping

Recognition of roles as an important factor in achieving a secure and satisfying identity has far-reaching effects and influences the way in which helping relationships are evaluated. It adds significance to the basic caring relationship as an enhancer of identity and throws light on the special needs of carers. Clarification of the connection between role-definition and outcome of help highlights the need for users to develop, and be enabled to develop, role and group identities which rather than focusing on their inadequacy and reinforcing their inferior position, empower them to cope with life. This brings into the open the considerable responsibility carried by those who are in a position to define the roles of others. It is because the designated role can influence collaborative situations that I now find myself wanting to replace the term 'user' by that of 'self-helper'.

Chapter 10
Working-Identity and Collaboration

Having seen how important roles are to the identity of the individual I look now at the identity that comes from working as a helper, in particular from belonging to a helping profession and working in a helping agency, and the bearing this has on collaboration.

The constituents of working-identity

Working identity stems from the *work-role* – that is, the particular duties to be carried out, often formulated in a written job description, and as currently interpreted by the agency and/or profession. This is the scripted part which the worker, like an actor, takes and interprets, fashioning out of it their own particular *working-role*. This is an individualised character role embodying certain activities and relational patterns. Workers bring to it aspects of their individual identity such as age, gender, cultural background, education, life experience, values, capabilities and personality. Personality includes motivation to help, ability to relate to people and the way in which anxiety is managed. Formal carers bring an identification with their agency, and practitioners with their profession also; there may be other relevant group affiliations, such as race or religion. Developments in society influence working-identity; the improvement of women's status has affected their confidence in professional roles, the freer style of personal relationships has had an impact on professional relationships, *'protocol'* – the behaviour patterns designed to maintain respect for status – being greatly diminished.

The working-identity of two people employed in an identical work-role may be very different and will affect their capacity to help in any particular situation. This is especially true where complex collaboration is needed. However much a professional persona may dominate a practitioner's working relationships, something of the individual identity will always come through and affect the relationship.

The value of a partly shared identity between helper and user can be important, and here self-help groups have something special to offer. Users sometimes feel that unless helpers have gone through the same experience they are not in a position to understand their situation. None the less parallel experience can often be a valid alternative; the experience of pain, loss, a broken relationship, being belittled, frustrated and set back constitute a common denominator in many distressing situations. Cultural background may be irrelevant in some helping situations and of great importance in others. Sometimes a user's situation cannot be understood sufficiently well for the appropriate help to be offered unless their cultural values and norms are understood, and this may require a practitioner who shares their cultural or religious affiliations. In a pluralist society a properly valued cultural identity is always important to a person's sense of identity and, whether a user or a faceworker, this will affect the way they function in a helping relationship.

Working-identity is seen to be a composite product. For practitioners, this means that the boundary of their working-identity always incorporates at least three major boundaries; those of the person, profession and agency.

The wish to help

Motivation springs from many sources. Some people are simply led into helping from a warm heart and energy surplus to the needs of their own family; others from political, religious or moral values. Others wish to help because they or their relatives have suffered, or because they have been particularly helped by someone and would like to do the same for others. Motivation may also be less conscious. People who within their personality have a particular need to make up for their feared destructive qualities may find helping a very positive way of dealing with their deep feelings of guilt. Some, from a sense of inner deprivation, wish to give to others what, consciously or unconsciously, they feel they lack in themselves. Besides the need to give, the need for power through the possession of special skills and access to resources, and the need for status and an improved self-image may also contribute to the wish to help.

Any or all of these motives can bring people into a helping-role. The wish for a career and earning capacity may lead them into a helping profession. Some faceworkers, whether filling a highly skilled or an unskilled job, may enter the helping services with no special helping motivation. From their natural humanity or through identification with the ethos of their profession or agency, they often carry out their work with great kindness and sensitivity.

Helping ethic

Mixed motivation need not be a hindrance in the helping-role. Power-seeking and enhancement of the self-image are basic human motivations and, so long as helpers' needs serve rather than interfere with the aims of helping they can be a useful spur to good work. Occasionally very real conflict of interest arises. For example, where the worker's financial or career needs conflict with the interests of the user. Personal ethic is of importance in containing egoistic tendencies. For practitioners this can be supported by their profession's ethical tradition and formal code of ethics. However if strong egoistic tendencies become incorporated in the ethos of a profession it will fail to help its members live up to their declared professional ideals and collaboration will inevitably suffer.

Working-identity is influenced by the other life commitments of a worker. A young worker may be idealistically enthusiastic in the wish to help, working long hours for little money, whereas an older person may be identified as much with the roles of earner and parent as with that of helper. Reconciling the interests of the various part-person identities within an individual identity and welding them into an integrated whole is an inherent human task. *Personal cohesion* depends on the integrative capacity of a worker's personality and on the values by which he or she lives. Linked to this there is a personal quality in working-identity which is difficult to define. It is a kind of personal authority which comes from neither professional nor hierarchic authority, a self-assurance which seems to derive from personal integrity, life experience and an accurate self-evaluation.

The ability to relate helpfully

People vary in their ability to relate easily to others. Some will fulfil their wish to help in impersonal ways, say, in administration, on committees, or in fund-raising. Within the helping professions there will be practitioners who are inept in personal relationships but extremely well-qualified where specialised knowledge and skill is required. Others will be naturally good at helping in a personalised relationship. Amongst these there are personal differences. Some relate more easily to an individual, others to a group, whether of individual users or a family; some are better with one category of user or trouble, some with another; not all workers are equally good with babies, adolescents and old people, nor feel equally at ease in working with those with handicaps, the dying or the mentally ill – aptitudes vary.

Whenever collaboration of more than a routine kind is required the helper needs the ability to listen and communicate, a wish to understand, and tolerance and respect for the other person. This includes recognising the user's capacity for self-help and, in secondary collaboration, valuing the other worker's particular contribution. Complementary to this is recognition by the helper of the limits of their own capacities. Often the primary task is of a practical nature, needing few words; then the helper's warmth and sympathy will be communicated in actions as much as in words. For those who are suffering from serious and long-term troubles this basic caring relationship may be the most important component of all the help they receive.

In specific work with relationships and feelings, the helper needs empathy

– the ability to identify with the situation of another and so obtain some emotional understanding of it, coupled with objectivity – the ability to remain outside a situation and evaluate it. This relational ability is determined by personality, but can be increased through training in relational skills. The wide variation between one worker and another in their ability to relate is of crucial importance to collaboration. If differences can be accepted, then those with relational ability can be used to the full, not only in primary, but also in secondary and participatory collaboration.

Professional identification

Most helpers find their way into a profession and an agency which suits their individual outlook and are then open to its influence. On the positive side professional and agency identifications lend strength to workers when carrying out difficult tasks. On the negative side they hinder workers from functioning at their best in collaborative situations because of various negative processes which take place at the professional and agency boundary.

Professional identity comes from the character role based on the possession of specialised skills and a particular role relationship with those who need them. The specific elements of the role are: professional aims, attitudes and values; categories of user and trouble served; methods practised (with their necessary skills, knowledge and theoretical base); and authority. These are embodied in the profession's training, qualification for membership, code of ethics and organisation; they are manifested in the practice of its members. Authority is an important constituent of professional identity. It stems from statutory power, level of expertise and training, power to access specific methods of help, the power of the profession's organisation, the power of the archetypal image and the status accorded by society in general and the user in particular.

Though professional identity is not static there seems to be a core-identity which remains stable and with which all members are able to identify. Around this lies an extended identity which is subject to modification as the result of widening fields of work, increased knowledge and skills, new methods of help, changes in attitudes and values or re-interpretation of old ones. A continuous process of development, internal discussion and external feedback shapes a profession's current identity. The result is a current general identity within which there will be many variations between different professional sub-groups, concerned with specialisms, attitudes and values.

Just as the individual needs to have a satisfying self-image, so a profession needs to establish, promote and protect a strong, cohesive and satisfying *professional image* with which its practitioners can identify. When a profession lacks this, its perceived identity will probably be varied and confused and the role-identity of its practitioners insecure, both of which will make secondary collaboration more difficult.

From the professional image a *professional stereotype* emerges. This is a generalised character role which embodies standard patterns of practice, values, comportment and attitudes to the user, members of the practitioner's own profession and other workers. If the stereotype incorporates rigid patterns of behaviour, it can dominate a practitioner's individual professional identity. The group influence to conform to the stereotype is strong, acting like a straitjacket which prevents an adaptive response. If the professional image can be one which gives value to individualism the stereotype is less likely to have a stultifying effect.

The perceived identity of a profession is based on the professional stereotype. It serves a useful purpose, as it enables people on first meeting to have some idea of what can be expected of the practitioner. For this reason it is important that it is clear and accurate. If, in an initial contact, practitioners are invested with a stereotype which is not too far away from their professional self-image, they may not be aware of it. If they sense a misfit, they probably try to differentiate themselves from a bad stereotype and may or may not do so from a good or idealised one.

Where a professional stereotype has close associations with an archetypal image it is possible for the practitioner, particularly if encouraged by the user, to fall into an archetypal identification and develop an inflated self-image. If practitioners are aware of carrying such an image they can, whilst differentiating themselves from it, often make deliberate use of the archetypal aura for the benefit of the user.

Although an idealised image may sometimes support practitioners in their work, it hinders complex collaborative relationships. The investment of a practitioner with a bad stereotype, which may lower working performance, has a similar effect. In all complex collaboration, stereotypes need to be shed, to allow the necessary individualised working relationships to develop.

Agency identification

The agency also needs a well-defined image with which its workers can identify and which can be accurately perceived by those outside it. Through its policy-making and management, the agency provides an administrative organisation, accountability and support structures, specific work-roles and priorities. Through the way in which it interprets and fulfils its purpose, an agency develops its own ethos – that is, its general atmosphere and style, including its attitude to users. These are all factors in providing a strong agency image. Identification with an agency means commitment to fulfilling its aims, a loyalty to the organisation and the workers in it. Practitioners may find themselves in a particular agency from necessity, but more often they have chosen one with aims, methods and an ethos with which they can easily identify, and an organisation in which they can feel at ease.

For faceworkers without a professional training the agency is likely to be their primary group identification; whereas for practitioners it may come second to professional identification, though not always so, particularly where the professional image is weak or ambiguous. The balance between professional and setting identifications varies considerably between one worker and another. For doctors, identification with the medical profession probably always outweighs that of setting. However, GPs who work in a health centre or have strong links with the local community and agencies may find the influence of setting modifying their professional identifications.

Community and institutional settings create different types of working-identity for members of the same profession. For example, the complicated and specialised structure and size of a hospital and the minimal requirements of, say, a family service unit provide very different settings for social workers. Many of the same skills will be needed in both but there will be considerable differences in the work-role, hierarchic structure, working procedures and comportment expected of the worker by users and other professions. It is not uncommon at a case conference for social workers from two such different settings to feel more closely identified with a member of another profession from their own agency or local community than with each other.

Practitioners do not always appreciate the need for a different working-identity in members of their own profession in another agency, judging them, for example, as too formal and rigid or too informal and easy-going. Since settings of different types attract practitioners of different types, certain patterns of behaviour may be reinforced, and the criticism may have validity. However in order to provide services well-adapted to the needs of users different degrees of informality in agencies is essential. For collaboration across such boundaries acceptance of differences is also essential.

Threats to working-identity

Loss of identity, a frightening experience, can be caused by loss of an important role or by damage to a group which is an important enhancer of the individual's sense of identity. Working-identity is threatened when practitioners feel that their role, profession or agency is endangered. This may be the result of change or of new developments leading to added power in the hands of other professionals or agencies. The strong reaction, indicating the strong need to protect working-identity, is illustrated in the following example.

A local group for mental health workers

A residential therapeutic community for people with mental health troubles had for some time been running its own agency liaison group, which met several times a year. In one meeting the view was put forward and strongly supported that there were other local workers concerned with mental health who did not come to this meeting because they had no connection with the agency, and that the meetings could be more useful if they served a wider range of workers. It was agreed that over and above the existing individual agency liaison groups a structure for a local network group for mental health workers was needed. As a result a committee was set up to organise an exploratory meeting for all potential members of such a group.

At the first meeting of the committee it was decided that the work would be expedited if a chairperson were appointed. The warden of the therapeutic community said it would be inappropriate for him to continue in this role, and suggested the director of the local MIND group. This was a developing agency which, whilst providing a number of useful projects, was perceived as empire-building. The suggestion did not meet with acclaim. A hospital social worker and an area social worker both indicated that they would be ready to serve as chairperson but neither backed the other. The CPN said nothing. It appeared that nobody was prepared to back anyone else. The MIND director then suggested a worker from a day centre, who declined, saying she was new in the area and had only come as a stand-in for her senior who was unable to attend. In the end it was agreed that the position of chair should rotate and that, for this meeting, it should still be taken by the warden of the therapeutic community. Plans for an open meeting for all local mental health workers were developed with some speed and the date for another committee meeting was arranged. The location became the subject of a second prolonged discussion. Four members offered their premises. Finally it was decided that the venue should also rotate.

About 60 people attended the open meeting and they decided to set up a local group for mental health. As in the committee meeting, there was a lengthy discussion on the chairmanship and the venue. Finally it was decided that those who had called the meeting should be elected as a steering group with no power except to arrange meetings, and at these meetings the chair should rotate between steering group members. Although various agencies offered a room for meetings free of charge, it was decided that the venue should be a church hall.

At the early steering group meetings, time was always spent on deciding who would be in the chair. This was thought to be inefficient and chairless meetings were tried. These were found to be equally time-consuming, no one liking to take the lead when it was necessary to bring the group to the point of making a decision. Only after a number of meetings did the steering group appoint a chairperson for six months, although the chair for meetings of the whole group continued to rotate.

An occasion arose in the steering group when a worker let fall the phrase: 'that agency with its tentacles ...' Someone drew attention to the appellation, and it opened up a discussion about their fears of expansionist tendencies in other agencies and the power-drive in other workers, vividly symbolised by the greedy octopus. These fears were found to be strong, nor did they lessen through discussion. However subsequently, they were recognised and referred to in a semi-joking manner.

The style of the group gradually developed into lunchtime meetings at approximately six-weekly intervals, with an attendance of between 15 and 20. Many came to the group only once or twice, but there was a core of regular attenders. Sandwiches were provided and the group sat in a circle, chaired in an informal way. Information was exchanged, followed by a short presentation and discussion. At the first few meetings practitioners presented the work of their agencies. Then the group began to discuss particular issues relating to collaboration, sometimes based on a theme, such as referrals or the combination of psychotherapy and drug treatment, sometimes a presentation of collaborative work carried out by two or more workers. No outside speakers were invited, the group deciding that it would use its own resources to work on collaborative issues. In time the group's aims were formulated in the following way: to offer an opportunity for workers in the field of mental health to get to know each other better, with a view to developing mutual trust; and to provide a forum for exchange of information and discussion of issues related to collaboration, with a view to improving practice.

There was always a division of interest between those who wished to pursue these aims through hearing more about other agencies and the methods of help available for specific problems, and those who wished to discuss their actual collaborative practice and go more deeply into the problems of collaborative relationships. All shared the wish to get to know other workers better and develop mutual trust. All seemed to agree that underneath the formal relationships of practitioners and those which were contained within the framework of defined procedures, as well as those without containing structure, there was little trust unless it had been developed on a personal basis. Finally the group settled for the discussion of collaborative relationships in which case- material would be brought. The group developed in this way because of the interest of a number of its members in the psychodynamic processes involved in collaboration and the presence of a group consultant. Thus constituted, the meetings were bound to arouse anxiety in members, in that their practice was exposed to the eyes of others outside their own agency. It was recognised that this was difficult but that it seemed the best way to understand the problems of collaboration between practitioners.

The group decided to provide occasional meetings to satisfy those who did not wish to be involved in specific discussion of practice, but this was only partially successful. The variety of needs of the workers serving the locality came out very clearly in this group, and the difficulty of adequately meeting all of them. When other similar groups for workers in mental health were set up in adjoining localities, they adopted different structures; meetings were less frequent and larger, presentations and discussions more formal and outside speakers invited.

Matters of difficulty between workers were often brought up, but some of the group's discussions were found to unite rather than divide workers from different professions and agencies. Common identifying factors which crossed these boundaries were brought to light; for instance, shared methods of therapeutic and counselling help, problems with difficult users, feelings of frustration and inadequacy, the assessment skills needed in generalist as opposed to specialist agencies, problems of referral, the problems in day and in-care settings of balancing the pressing need for taking in new users with the need for adequate time to make plans for those leaving the setting, problems of handover and managing transitional stages for users.

Regular attenders, and particularly those who served for a time on the steering committee, said that they developed greater mutual trust as a result of face-to-face contact and open exchanges; increased understanding of the strengths, limitations and problems of other professions and agencies; a clearer appraisal of the strengths and limitations of their own skills and their agency's functions; a clearer idea of the causes of mistrust and deeper understanding of collaborative problems. This had resulted in less uncertainty-in-role, greater tolerance and fellow-feeling for other workers and a better use of other agencies.

Identification with the group was never strong in comparison with agency identification. On one occasion workers from a voluntary agency asked for the group's support because its borough grant was to be cut and closure threatened. In the discussion that followed it became evident that although everybody valued this agency and did not wish it to close, when widespread cuts in funding were in progress competition between agencies was real, and practitioners could only be concerned for their own agency, unless its position was totally secure.

Looking at the development of this group it can be seen that in the initial stages there was considerable fear that workers from other agencies would try and acquire power in order to use the group for their own unspecified ends. Once the group had formed, a structure was established which contained these fears and made it possible for a shared identity gradually to develop. Concern for helping those with mental health needs in the locality was the common denominator and, on this basis, the group was able to consolidate, although there were many underlying tensions. Cohesion in the steering group, as a result of open discussion, was of great importance in providing a strong core-group. In the group as a whole there was sufficient cohesion to contain the anxiety aroused when professional and agency rivalries were brought into the open.

It is difficult to assess how valid these fears were; certainly, some agencies were developing whilst others remained static. The problem of competition for funds was spoken about openly and seemed to be accepted as inevitable. Other fears seemed to have a less rational basis. They centred on the expansionist tendencies in other agencies, symbolised by the grasping octopus, and on role-insecurity when presenting work to an interagency group. An interesting example of the fears aroused by agency development was afforded by one particular group discussion.

A new agency I

Some years after the group for mental health started, a new psychiatric unit, with in-, out- and day care facilities, was opened at the local district hospital. This development had been much needed and strongly supported by all local agencies. Those in charge of the unit had organised a number of agency liaison meetings before and after it was opened, in order to keep local workers informed and to enlist their co-operation in the unit's early development. Although many members of the group for mental health had participated in these meetings, the steering group decided to ask some practitioners in the unit to present its work at a group meeting.

A number of the agency's workers came and described the present services and plans for future development. There was considerable overlap with existing day care, counselling and therapeutic services provided by the agencies of members in the group. These agencies had been used extensively by the psychiatrists who had held out-patient clinics at the hospital before the new unit was opened. Although everyone knew that an overall increase of services had been needed, the presentation met with a cool reception. Questions turned on how much the hospital would continue to refer to existing agencies. Someone suggested that it would now only refer on the rather hopeless cases. Very considerable unease and rivalry was apparent. Finally someone said that perhaps there would not be enough patients to go round. Once this fear was articulated there seemed to be an easing of tension, and the discussion took a more positive turn, looking at the important differences between similar services when they were provided in health or social care settings and how this could improve the overall service.

In succeeding meetings there were discussions as to the overlapping purposes served by the local network group and the liaison meetings held at the hospital. The basic differences between an agency-centred· network and a locality-centred network were clarified. It became apparent that the position of the hospital practitioners was very different in the two groups. Most of them were prepared to put more effort into their own liaison meetings, but they wanted at least one from their team to take an active part in the local network group. This seemed appropriate in terms of time-efficiency, pointing to the need for a specialised collaborative role to be carried by one or two practitioners in an agency.

Fear for agency survival seems to have been manifest in the remark that 'there might not be enough patients to go round', by and large an unrealistic anxiety, comparable to that symbolised by the grasping octopus. There is an irrational quality about such reactions which seems to be common in workers who are closely identified with their agency. Group reactions are known to be more primitive than those of individuals, and here it can be seen how they militate against collaboration.

On an individual basis, working-identity is threatened by comparison of competence in a particular skill or field of help. *Competence* is the result of ability, training and experience. Able faceworkers with experience but no formal training frequently suffer role-insecurity when collaborating with trained workers. This was clear in the volunteers at the MIND centre (Chapter 8) but it also applies to paid workers in responsible positions with better qualified workers under them, and to senior practitioners if those accountable to them are recently trained and conversant with new trends in their profession.

Role-insecurity

The anxiety people feel about their performance or relationships in a particular role is described by the terms *role-insecurity*. It may result from either threats to working identity, as described above, uncertainty-in-role or personal anxiety.

Uncertainty-in-role is felt by faceworkers when they are unsure of what they are doing. It is not so much that their working-identity is threatened, as that they give it a poor rating because of a sense of inadequacy, which may stem from a number of causes. They may be dealing with a formidable situation for which adequate solutions have not been found or that demand resources beyond those which are available, whether human, material or institutional. Alternatively they may lack the necessary competence or authority to match the task. Sometimes the work-role has been ill-defined, so that faceworkers are unsure of the content and limits of their work. If there is uncertainty in the agency as to its proper function or its future development, the resulting group uncertainty is likely to be experienced by its practitioners as their own insecurity.

Personal anxiety has different causes according to the helpers' core-personality structure. Some people are thrown by being in a situation which is confused or out of control; others set themselves an unduly high standard of achievement, and feel pressured, not only by their own expectations, but by those of the user and other workers. Personal anxiety also arises from the reactivation of anxieties from the past. They may come from conscious recollection of unhappy experiences; or from unconscious or semi-conscious fears belonging to early childhood, which can easily be touched off by distressing or frightening situations.

The feelings which are evoked in workers as a result of role-insecurity can usually only be spoken about in discussions where trust is well established, and some of my examples have been taken from such situations. I have found that when these feelings are described, although they normally operate at a covert level, other workers are quite familiar with them. Tolerance of role-insecurity depends on the personal constituent in working-identity. The stronger the sense of personal identity underlying the role, the greater the ability to experience and tolerate role-insecurity – the converse is also true. When it cannot be tolerated, the faceworker inevitably resorts to a defensive process.

Chapter 11
Working-Identity: The Defended Position

In the previous chapter I showed why it is so important to practitioners to feel secure in their working-role. It is natural that people sometimes feel insecure when engaged in difficult tasks and relationships. However there are ways to increase role-security, some of which improve and others which detract from the practitioner's capacity to help. In this chapter I look more particularly at the latter, illustrating some of the processes by which a secure working-identity is maintained at the expense of collaborative relationships.

Coping and defending

Working stress is the internal tension that results either from emotional reactions to normally stressful tasks and responsibilities or to exceptional situations. Stress in faceworkers is inevitable because of their difficult tasks, heavy responsibilities and the distressing situations they face. While working they must control emotion and contain anxiety. The way in which people manage their reactions to stress is an important constituent of their working-identity.

Coping methods include the personal methods of individual faceworkers, the group methods of professions and other groups of faceworkers, and the structural methods of professions and agencies. They may be either *concurrent*, those that operate during the stressful situation, or *sequential*, those which cope with stress after the event. For most practitioners, *concurrent coping methods* function automatically, in response to the situation. For instance the restriction of their view of the user to the presenting trouble, in order to limit awareness of distress whilst coping with the immediate situation. Or the suppression of feeling when emotional reactions in the worker are strong and their expression would be unhelpful, or when practical action requires total attention. These are *coping mechanisms*.

Practitioners have their own *personal coping methods* but can also make use of those belonging to their profession. Because groups are systems made up of people, they are able to incorporate in their structure the coping mechanisms used by individuals. These may become institutionalised in a standard form, and are then available to individual practitioners to adopt as

119

their own. *Professional coping methods* are essential to the support of practitioners, the purpose being to foster efficiency in the fulfilment of tasks. In addition the agency's routines and procedures, whilst designed for efficiency, frequently also serve to contain reactions to stress, constituting *structural coping methods*.

Sequential coping methods range from an informal talk with a friend or colleague, to a regular formal session, either for a group or an individual. A suitable place and time is provided in which work can be reviewed, anxieties and difficult or distressing emotions shared and discussed with others. This process, as well as alleviating stress, often enables faceworkers to develop personal responses which are better adapted to the situations they have to face.

The primary purpose of coping methods is to help a faceworker function optimally in a temporary situation of stress. However, the same processes may be used for other ends. *Defensive processes* are aimed at protecting an insecure role-identity at all times, not only in times of immediate stress and, instead of helping good practice, they work against it. When an essential coping mechanism is made use of in this way, it then becomes a *defence mechanism* – an automatic and largely unconscious response to a situation, designed to prevent the experience of anxiety. Factors determining the need for faceworkers to use them are: the level of stability of their sense of identity; the degree of stress to which they are subject in their work; and whether sequential coping methods are available for handling stress in a mature way. If they are not available, then normal stress can be compounded by unnecessary role-insecurity.

Defences which have been developed at the individual level can be taken over by a group and may eventually become institutionalised into the group's structure and mode of functioning. The theory of *institutionalised group defences* was developed by Isabel Menzies Lyth in 1959, as a result of her study of nurses in a large teaching hospital (see Further Reading). Here she shows how the anxieties raised by their tasks may reactivate anxieties of childhood, thus increasing the need for coping structures, if strong defences are to be avoided. She illustrates how the profession has developed institutionalised defences which have become built into the nurses' patterns of functioning. She stresses how defensive patterns are unsatisfactory because, although anxiety is to some extent contained, 'true mastery of anxiety by deep working-through and modification is seriously inhibited'. The institutionalised defences of any profession will hinder its practitioners from developing less stressed and more mature attitudes to the inevitable anxieties of their work.

Certain *personal defence mechanisms* operate through a self-contained process within the individual. For instance, repression of emotion may lead to symptoms such as headaches or other functional disorders, perhaps necessitating sick-leave. Other defensive patterns, instead of being contained inside the personal system, make use of the group system, which will then function badly, and others operate at the individual's or group's boundary. These are the ones which are particularly harmful to collaborative relationships.

Here I am not concerned with the defences against anxiety that individuals use in their ordinary life, but with those they use in their working-role, whether personal or institutionalised in the professional or agency system. The following examples illustrate common defensive processes. They have been drawn from discussions in which practitioners were working to understand collaborative problems.

Withdrawal defences

Defences I

> **A** teacher, who specialised in helping children with reading difficulties, said: 'The parents of many of my pupils need help but I have not the time to see them, so they have to go without'.

> A GP said: 'In principle I believe in a holistic approach to my patients, but I am not so arrogant as to think that I am able to carry out all the work that this would entail. I cannot therefore put such an approach into practice in the way I would like for my patients'.

Both practitioners were using the defence of *withdrawal* coupled with a *denial of reality*. The teacher spoke as if she had all the skills necessary for helping parents, although she had neither experience nor training in this work. The GP, whilst recognising that he did not have the necessary skills, seemed to deny the reality that there were other practitioners who did have them. Both showed genuine concern for the users of their services but here, by withdrawing behind their professional boundaries, they failed them.

Such a defensive process protects an unrealistic self-image and maintains a false sense of role-security. If the teacher had been open to referring to another practitioner, she would have had to face the fact that she was unable to offer all the help necessary, not only for lack of time but also for lack of skill. If the GP had started to refer on, he would have had to accept that there were other people with the skills he lacked. Both practitioners would have had to modify an omnipotent aspect of their professional self-image. Such a process would have meant facing role-insecurity before their collaborative practice could be developed.

These two examples of withdrawal, linked with some denial of reality, show how the defence prevents users getting the help they need even when the need is recognised. Such collaborative non-events seldom come to light, but are none the less common for that. There seems to be a deep-rooted attitude in both users and faceworkers that they should always be able to cope with their own emotions without assistance, and with the emotional troubles of others without special training. In many discussions, practitioners have said that they experience no problem in referring on for general or specialised medical help but, when it is a question of referring for counselling or psychotherapy of some kind, they feel it indicates a failure on their part and that they should have been able to handle such problems themselves. Although this is known to be a common reaction in users, it is not so well recognised that faceworkers can feel the same way. Referral-on seems to constitute a considerable blow to their professional self-image, so that defences are used to avoid role-insecurity.

It is not only the basic helping professions that have a resistance to referring on in the sphere of relational work. Those with specialised relational skills have a similar problem, when the use of a more experienced practitioner or a different type of therapy is indicated.

Defences II

In a discussion including individual and group psychotherapists with various types and levels of training, a social worker who was also an experienced group therapist said: 'I find it easy to recognise those with less skill than myself, who might well refer cases to me, but it is not so easy to recognise those with more skill, who might be able to help certain people better than I can'.

Later in the discussion a consultant psychiatrist said: 'I have trained as both an individual and group analyst, so when it comes to looking at family therapy, I have to choose between one of the following positions: because of the qualifications I already have, I can do it; or, I have not got the skills, but they are not worth having, because family therapy is useless anyway – the 'sour grapes syndrome'; or, I have not got the skills and I know that family therapy is of some use, so either I must learn how to do it or I must be able to assess when it would be helpful and be ready to refer on'.

The *sour grapes defence* is designed to avoid experiencing envy, by devaluing the object which has provoked it, thus maintaining role-security. Recognition of the defence means that it is not adopted. The illustration, although taken from a specialised field, describes very clearly a common process that take place in many practitioners. As happens in many developing spheres of practice, there is a wide range of competence and little agreement concerning the measurement of skills. This encourages comparison, envy and rivalry, and is likely to cause much role-insecurity with consequent recourse to defensive processes.

Transboundary defences

Two of the commonest defensive processes making use of the professional or agency boundary are the *displacement defence* and what I call the *downing defence*. In the following example both defences are operating, and professional and agency boundaries are both involved.

Defences III

In a small meeting concerned with collaboration in mental health the question had been raised concerning the value of informal agencies, with reference to a particular drop-in centre run by the social services department, which people could attend without going through any formal assessment procedure. The centre was run by a trained worker, but largely staffed by untrained personnel. In the discussion some members of the group said that this informal method of help could, for certain types of disturbed person, be more beneficial than the hospital psychiatric services. A psychiatrist agreed with them and went further, in advocating greater involvement of people from ordinary life situations. He described how he had contact with an employer concerning a patient whom he feared might commit suicide. When this patient had failed his last appointment, the psychiatrist had phoned the employer. A social worker queried whether he should have had this contact without permission from his patient, implying that he had become over-involved in the case. Another psychiatrist from the same hospital immediately took the discussion back to the informal helping services. He said that he acted as supervisor to a group of volunteers working in a mental health project. They were very committed and he admired their enthusiasm and the way in which they gave freely of their time. However he wondered about their motivation and thought many of them were over-identified with the people they were trying to help.

By talking about the volunteers whose work he supervised, he drew attention away from his colleague, deflecting his own potentially hostile criticism on to workers outside the group boundary. This displacement defence is often used to preserve cohesion and harmony within agencies, departments or teams. It defends workers against the role-insecurity which arises from hostility within a group, by directing it elsewhere. At the same time, through interweaving the two themes of unqualified worker and over-involvement, *inadequacy* is also placed outside the boundary of the discussion group. Thus the greater competence of the well-trained worker and the formal helping services is firmly established in relation to less trained workers and more informal services. In this process the unacceptable attribute is projected on to another worker or agency which is 'downed' so that the first worker or agency may be correspondingly 'upped'. This defence protects against role-insecurity when the worker's self-image as a competent practitioner is under threat.

The downing defence might be thought a comparatively harmless process provided that the downed workers are absent and do not suffer personally. In fact it militates against good practice in general and collaborative practice in particular. In the above example, it deflected the whole group from pursuing a useful line of discussion on confidentiality in relation to the user, to which members of various professions would have contributed, and which might have led to greater understanding of their different attitudes to helping. It also resulted in a subjective and unchallenged assessment of the work of the denigrated agency that could detract from its use by other members of the group.

These same defences together with others are illustrated in the following description of collaborative difficulties between two social work agencies. The example shows how, as the result of considerable working over of areas of tension, recognition of the defensive processes that were operating at the agency interface was followed by development of mutual understanding and trust, which ultimately enabled defences to be dropped and change to take place.

Referral problems I

I was asked by two social workers to help them with a problem of referrals between their agencies, which they had tried unsuccessfully to resolve themselves. Both were skilled and committed workers so that, in the process of working on the problem, we went more deeply than usual into the hidden hindrances that were operating between the two agencies. This piece of work was undertaken some years ago and since then there have been changes in both agencies and in certain social work attitudes. However, the negative processes so clearly illustrated here still operate at the boundaries between agencies, and between departments or teams within an agency. Thus, although some of the details in the illustration may be less applicable today the relational processes are as relevant as ever.

Brenda was the head of a voluntary agency which provided counselling for individuals and families, and which was staffed by qualified social workers, experienced in psychotherapeutic work. The agency's catchment area covered a wide range of socio-economic groups. Within this area, Jill was team-leader of the intake team of a social services department area office, which served a neighbourhood with multiple inner-city problems. The intake team saw all new referrals and the number of applicants for help could not be easily controlled. Following the initial interview the team operated priorities for regulating the inflow of their clients. High priority was given to statutory work and to urgent cases. Some of these were referred immediately to long-term teams in the area office, others taken on for short-term work, i.e. a period of up to three months. Of the clients with low priority who could not be adequately helped in the initial interview, some were advised where else to apply and their case closed. Other cases were kept open, in order that the worker might seek an alternative agency to help them. Jill had a strong commitment to referral-on, but there was little time for this work. Brenda's agency was one of those used but despite discussion Jill felt uncertain of their criteria for accepting cases.

Both workers were concerned at the time wasted by failed referrals, and the intake team as a whole was said to feel very negative towards the counselling agency. This agency's intake procedure took about three weeks. The referral was first considered by the whole team; if accepted, a worker was appointed for the initial interview, the result of which was discussed at a subsequent team meeting. A decision was then taken and if the case was accepted a worker was allocated. A referrer was expected to provide an informative written report, to have clarified any previous involvement of other agencies and prepared their client for the transfer. This procedure was primarily designed to select clients who would be sufficiently motivated and integrated to be helped within the agency's structure of regular appointments. Although their clients came more often from other sources of referral, some people seen by the area social work office could be helped by the agency provided the transfer could be effected. However, workers in the area office intake team resented the referral requirements, thinking them unrealistic, if not unnecessary.

The two workers and I met on my premises with the intention of planning a joint meeting of their two teams. We started by clarifying the current procedures, as outlined above. This was followed by a discussion in which it became apparent that, though there was much disagreement, they shared one view in common: there must be change, and this must be in the other agency, change in their own being out of the question.

In this first meeting, not only were the different positions of the two workers starkly exposed, but we experienced a wholly unexpected intensity of hostility. It seemed out of the question to think of getting the two teams together until some of the problems had been worked through between their two senior workers. We met four times at approximately monthly intervals. These meetings were hard going but a strong group identity developed, enabling us to clarify facts and understand some of the difficult feelings involved.

The second meeting began by sharing the shock reactions we had experienced after the first one, and this immediately evoked fellow-feeling. Each worker said that she felt her situation had been misunderstood and her point of view unheard. This common experience strengthened the bond and both became more open to hearing what the other wished to communicate. Although the facts outlined above had been known, much about the conditions of work and the functions and values of each agency was either not known or not fully appreciated.

Certain specific misunderstandings emerged. For example, the area office had been extremely short-staffed for a time, and cases had been referred to the counselling agency which would have been better handled within the social services department. Because Jill had not conveyed their predicament clearly enough, the counselling agency's response had been inappropriately critical. This only highlighted a long-standing situation of poor communication between the two workers. There had been remarkably little feedback concerning failed referrals and consequently little opportunity to learn from mistakes; but even more damaging had been the hangover of unresolved ill-feeling which continued to fester. Details of failed referrals were brought up, some from long ago but as fresh as if they had only just occurred.

Differences between the agencies – their function, priorities and methods of work – gradually became clearer. Jill described how she and her team valued a quick response to whatever personal troubles or social problems their clients might present, with adaptability and resourcefulness as the keynote for seeking solutions. Because of the impossibility of regulating the inflow of cases, time given to any one client was partly determined by the need to respond concurrently to other clients, varying in number and urgency. By contrast, the counselling agency was able to regulate its inflow. Their workers gave value to a thorough assessment based on comprehensive information and a long initial interview. On this basis the team decided the most appropriate help. Methods offered included both general counselling and 'in-depth' work. An assessment of the client's personality and situation was required and, on occasion, a psychiatrist's report. It became clear that the functions and constraints of each agency had a considerable influence on the kind of social work practised within it. There was a strong tendency in each worker to assume that methods appropriate to her own agency should be relevant to the other with little or no modification. This assumption seemed inappropriate to two such experienced workers and slowly it emerged that their views were influenced by unrecognised emotions.

The attitudes polarised on the axis of 'long' and 'short' term work. Jill considered the counselling agency workers, with their relatively small caseload, to be overprotected, precious, doctrinaire and 'often irrelevant to the needs of most clients'. Brenda judged intake workers as muddled, superficial, over-involved and 'always rushing about'. The simplistic and intransigent quality of the comments pointed towards an irrational element in what was presented as a rational assessment of the other agency.

Gradually both workers felt sufficiently safe and committed to the task to risk abandoning their defensive positions. Each then described feelings of envy. Jill envied long-term workers their opportunity to carry out in-depth work with well-motivated clients; Brenda envied short-term workers the possibility of setting limited goals and seeing a case through to its conclusion.

The sour grapes defence contributed strongly to the denigration of the other agency. Later it came out that intake workers were also envious of the long-term workers in their own area office and that for the sake of maintaining good relationships inside their agency, without realising it, this feeling was displaced outside their agency boundary, thus compounding the negative feelings already directed towards the counselling agency.

The two workers began to share the doubts they had about the quality and effectiveness of their own and their teams' social work practice. Brenda said that she and her workers feared they would be 'lumbered' with cases which they would be unable to help but would feel they could not close; a hidden factor in their selective intake. Jill feared lest her team should carry too many low priority cases. Hidden factors in her unwillingness to prepare cases for referral-on were her fears that, as a result of insufficient skill, her workers would either inadvertently form a relationship which would militate against transfer, or else, without deliberate intent, bring this about in order to avoid taking on more urgent and more difficult cases. Anxiety in both teams arising from doubts about the quality of their practice had been partially avoided by the downing defence, in which the unacceptable element of inadequate practice had been split off and projected on to the other agency. Cross-projections developed easily between these two agencies because their professional style and values polarised so readily.

Jill then described how she and her team experienced themselves as 'the poor relation' of the long-term workers, in whatever agency the latter might be working. Social casework in the past had placed a high value on long-term work but intake workers did not hold this view. However it seemed that they were still influenced by it and thus deemed their work inferior to that of the long-term workers. It seemed that they were open to being used by long-term workers to carry a 'bad' image in order that the morale of the others might be maintained. It became clear that problems between the intake team and the long-term teams in the area office had not been sorted out because they had never been brought into the open. Denial of these problems had led to displacement of the intake team's negative feelings outside the agency.

Jill described how Brenda's workers, when receiving a referral, would sometimes require a great deal more information than had been provided. She described how although the questions they asked seemed valid they had somehow left her intake workers feeling not only frustrated but inferior, useless and hopeless. We began to see in this 'over-questioning' by the worker receiving the referral a largely unconscious process, not only for putting off acceptance of a daunting case but also for avoiding the recognition that the receiving worker might not be able to cope with such a case and the consequent feelings of uselessness. This defence was effected at the expense of the referring worker, who was used as a repository for these unacceptable feelings of inadequacy, and who accepted this function.

Hidden processes on the part of the referring workers also came to light. Without deliberate intent but because of the strong need to pass on work, they did not always disclose a particular anxiety they might have about the case; for instance, the possibility that a member of the family might be liable to violence. A suspicion of being manipulated was aroused in the receiving worker, sometimes during discussion of the referral, sometimes when further facts came to light after the case had been transferred. This fed the existing lack of trust.

Although we had uncovered and worked on a number of difficulties and, in the third meeting, Jill outlined some modifications she had made, the point of deadlock remained; each required the other to change certain procedures and each was convinced that it was impossible for her agency to do so. Tension was high, defeat seemed imminent. We agreed that in the subsequent meeting we should consider whether to end. This fourth meeting began with a long discussion about rigid and flexible styles of social work practice which, when brought back to the two agencies themselves, produced a long and heavy silence. Brenda broke it by saying that if there were to be change on her side, her team must participate. She suggested that Jill and I should meet with them.

Throughout our four meetings we had been aware that Brenda came from a close-knit group of experienced workers who participated in decision-making; whereas the members of Jill's team changed more frequently, were less experienced, less concerned with decision-making and general policy. Because of this, feedback to the two teams during the course of our meetings had been very different. Now it seemed right that Brenda's team should be brought in to the discussion.

We had two meetings with the team, on their own premises. We worked over the same themes but more quickly. Afterwards Brenda said that she had been very nervous, fearing that Jill would be strongly attacked, but the discussions had proved direct without being destructive. Equally Jill feared the reaction which Brenda would get when we subsequently met with the intake team. Here, in fact, there was a strong attack on the counselling agency and its methods. However after working over difficulties and bad feelings, in the third meeting Jill enabled her team to recognise that they too had their deficiencies. She said that sometimes they had mistakenly accepted cases that should have been refused and had then tried to get rid of them by referring them on, almost inevitably courting a negative response and criticism. Accepting this self-criticism caused the team to reach a deep 'low', no longer being able to avoid the experience of depression by projecting their inadequacy into the other agency and condemning it there. The silence that followed seemed very depressed, and had the same quality as that in the last meeting we had had as a threesome. In a similar way, it was out of the depressed silence that a new and practical suggestion emerged. This was for a series of intake team meetings to be attended by Brenda, in which possible cases for referral-on would be discussed very soon after the client's first interview.

I shall not go into the details of these meetings except to say that although they were approached cautiously there was considerable goodwill; the referral process began to work better and the issues of procedure which had appeared so intractable ceased to be a stumbling-block. In addition, the counselling agency began to look at the process of contract-making with their clients as a means of creating time limits to their work.

This example illustrates three transboundary defences using different projective processes. The displacement defence is used to shift hostile feelings felt towards workers inside an agency on to workers in another agency in order to avoid internal agency conflict, and thus defend against an insecure group identity. The downing defence is used to avoid self-criticism through the projection of bad practice into another agency. In the helping services, fertile ground in which these two defensive processes can flourish is usually readily available. This means that if an agency does not sort out, or at least face and contain, its internal problems concerning hostile relationships and levels of practice, it is liable to damage its external relationships with some of the agencies with which it needs to collaborate.

The operation of a further transboundary defence is also illustrated. I name it the '*drowning defence*' because the process calls to mind the image of one person being pushed right under so that the other persons's head may remain above water. It is a transboundary process in which, unlike the downing defence, the two parties, whether individuals or groups, are both participating and must be in direct communication. This defence is illustrated in the above example in the description of the feelings of utter uselessness that were experienced by the intake worker after being over-questioned by the counselling worker. In their conversation the intake worker seems to have internalised and identified with the feelings of inadequacy which the counselling worker had split off and was getting rid of by the process of projection. In this way one worker succeeds in preserving a sense of competence at the expense of another, who allows themself to be put into the position of carrying an exaggerated feeling of incompetence. Although to be vulnerable to such a process the latter person must already contain within themselves some equivalent feeling to which the projection becomes attached, the feelings subsequently experienced are no longer theirs alone.

Some people are more vulnerable than others to this process of internalising the projected feelings of another. It occurs at the personal boundary, but it affects the group which the person represents or with which that person is identified. Between the above two agencies it had operated through a number of personal relationships but its effects were experienced by both groups.

It is apparent how these two closely related defences of downing and drowning had enabled each team of workers to avoid looking critically at its own practice, and had enabled the counselling workers to avoid experiencing their own feelings of inadequacy whilst causing the intake workers to feel irrationally inadequate and resentful. These defences thus effectively prevented internal change and caused a worsening of the interagency relationship.

Role-definition, as described in Chapter 9, can sometimes closely resemble the drowning defence. In fact it may act as an unrecognised institutionalised defence, deeply embedded in social custom. An individual or group in a power position can use it to define modal role relationships in a way that serves as a defence against an insecure role-identity, at the expense of the weaker party, who then carries the inferior qualities. In the case of faceworkers this is usually a sense of inadequacy but, in other situations, it could be other despised qualities. This can take place in any individual or group relationship: between a helper and user; between workers and a particular group of users; and between one group of workers and another.

Fragmenting defences

A narrow viewing-point focusing down on only one or a very few aspects of the user's situation is likely to be time-efficient and lead to optimum help when the trouble is straightforward or when the urgency of one of its aspects clearly takes precedence. In such cases it would be inappropriate to view the user as a whole person. However, when the trouble is complex focusing on one aspect only may result in failure to assess the situation adequately and, hence, failure to provide optimum help. It may also be harmful, through causing unnecessary fragmentation of the wholeness of an individual or family user.

Such a narrow viewing-point may be the result of an inadequate helping approach, but it may be due to converting a useful procedure and coping mechanism into a defence mechanism. This I term *perceptual fragmentation*. The user's situation can easily touch off in the faceworker reactions of distress, inadequacy or hostility, which frequently lead to role-insecurity. The faceworker is enabled to shut off these emotional reactions by ignoring the emotional aspects of a user's situation or only seeing them as a trouble which can be dealt with by physical, material or environmental methods of help. It inevitably means that the possible causal connection between the user's emotions and troubles is denied. Perceptual fragmentation may also be adopted by a worker as a defence against role-insecurity arising from lack of a certain skill. For example a practitioner who is highly skilled in certain areas may lack relational skills and defend against recognising this by failing to perceive relevant feelings in the user.

The aim of personal and social integration can be adversely affected by the procedures, routines and task distribution of professional and agency organisation, particularly in any form of in-care. In certain situations the rigid performance of routines and the allocation of different tasks to different workers is necessary, perhaps for guarding against mistakes which could be dangerous, or perhaps for providing workers with a useful coping method. In other circumstances they may be serving as a defensive method by constricting personal relationships and thus reducing the experience of feelings.

This I term *procedural fragmentation* because it is the way in which tasks are organised which hinders workers from relating to the user as an individual. Whilst diminishing role-insecurity, it often prevents fulfilment of the caring role in the way most helpful to the user and most satisfying to the helper. Menzies Lyth, in the paper already mentioned, describes the way this can affect the nurse's relationship to the patient and its effect on the nurse. Job satisfaction is reduced because the worker's potential contribution to the helping-task is not utilised to the full. If such a defensive process has become institutionalised within agency organisation, it is difficult for the individual worker to avoid its effects.

Organisational defences

Collaboration across the divide between the agencies of health and social care has particular problems because, having developed independently for so long, basic differences have been built into agency structures so firmly that modification is difficult. A simple example is the different hours of district nurses and social workers for starting work and for being in their office for phone calls, often making contact difficult. Lack of understanding in practitioners of organisational differences leads to an unnecessary mismatch between expectations of another agency and its performance. However, I think that complaints of this nature are often used as a defence against looking at deeper collaborative difficulties, whose tackling requires considerable motivation. In the example of the two social work agencies the organisational problems melted away when the deeper difficulties were faced.

The effects of defences on collaboration

Because defensive processes function in such a covert way they are difficult to observe directly, but the above examples give some idea of how they operate in working situations. I have focused particularly on those processes which make use of individual and group boundaries since it is here that they have such a negative effect on collaboration. The aim of these defences is to maintain a secure identity but whilst doing this they jeopardise the equally basic need for a satisfying identity. They inevitably restrict relationships and hinder development of personal potential so that in the long run they work against individual and group well-being. Defence mechanisms based on withdrawal preclude contact with others or render the relationship formal and superficial. Those based on denial of reality, whether linked with an omnipotent attitude or with a denigrating one, prevent a reality-based relationship. Those based on projection may prevent contact or, through distorting perceived identity, limit and distort relationships. Projective defences which cause the other party to internalise a negative projection, and fragmenting defences, in addition to distorting relationships, also diminish or harm the identity of the one on the receiving end.

All the defence mechanisms described can be incorporated into the identity of a group making them readily available for use by its members, and they may be actually inculcated along with other identifying features of the group. Indeed, the structuring of professional practice may be partly geared to maintaining such institutionalised defences as well as to developing the practitioner's full capacity for helpful working relationships. The difficulty here is that defence mechanisms are frequently developed out of the coping mechanisms which are essential to professional practice.

Through the examples given in this chapter I have attempted to demonstrate the significance of institutionalised as well as personal defences for maintaining a secure working-identity, and their potentially damaging effects. These are fourfold: critical appraisal of practice is curtailed; the development of a well-adapted response to stressful situations is impeded; all types of collaborative relationship are restricted; fear of change is increased, through fear of losing a well-established defence. The beneficial effect of discarding defences and facing the consequent role-insecurity is shown in the example of referral between two social work agencies.

The operation of defences disturbs collaborative practice, but to disturb defences threatens security. This is a formidable block to bringing about change and development in collaborative practice. Since the need for security is a strong and valid motivating force not easily overridden, the question is whether methods can be found to enable faceworkers to maintain a secure working-identity without damaging their transboundary relationships.

Chapter 12
Professional and Agency Identity: The Separatist Position

In the previous chapter I described hindrances to collaboration resulting from defensive processes. In this chapter, I look at those arising from a separatist outlook. Again this results from the misuse of a positive aspect of professional and agency functioning.

If faceworkers are to provide optimum help they need to operate from a firm *working-base* – the physical, organisational and psychological position from which their working-role is carried out. For this to be well-established, they need to know what their working-role covers, what authority it gives them, the current position and priorities of their agency and what it has sanctioned them to say and do on its behalf. They need to feel sure of the support of their profession and/or agency in what they are undertaking, and to be provided with adequate methods for coping with work stress. The working-base will be strengthened if workers also have a strong *identity-base* – a sense of knowing who they are in their working-role. This results from identification with their profession and/or agency, its aims and methods. It is strengthened if the worker feels part of a group of like-minded colleagues who, whatever their profession, share the same helping-approach and attitudes towards their work. This provides a secure place where they can feel at ease, speak freely, let off steam and exchange ideas, and where their identity can be validated through the support of others. Workers in large agencies can usually find such an identity-base. It is the principal workers in local voluntary agencies who most commonly experience the lack of it, through lack of a peer group, however supportive their committee may be.

A firm working-base will foster creativity and confidence in the face-worker, and is especially important in complex collaboration. Here, it enables faceworkers to contribute their particular view, arrived at from the *sectional viewing-point* of their profession and agency. Every profession and agency needs to have its own view of a particular situation, grounded in its special contribution to the provision of help. This provides the practitioner with a *sectional view* which can then be integrated with those of other faceworkers in order to arrive at a composite whole. In the context of a collaborative enterprise, it is then possible clearly to define the potential input from the various professions and/or agencies.

When the sectional viewing-point is over-restricted, owing to a limited helping-approach, it leads to MEC blindness, the faceworker being unaware of the need for collaboration. Like coping-methods, the sectional view can be used in a negative way and deteriorate into *separatism*: the pursuit of sectional ends for the self-interest of the organisation, profession or worker, rather than for the provision of an optimum service to the user. This chapter looks at some of the consequences of separatism.

Insufficient understanding of other professions

Disciplines – the body of knowledge and skills of the various professions – draw on a wide range of academic disciplines, including the natural sciences, psychology and sociology. These inevitably provide their own particular viewing-point from which to observe any situation and a framework within which to formulate thoughts about what has been perceived. These frameworks are an important element in core professional identity, being incorporated in basic training. Whilst forming valid elements in the boundaries between professions they are often negatively divisive. When trained to conceptualise in one way it is not easy to appreciate another way of viewing the same situation. The basic assumptions of a practitioner's own frame of reference are taken for granted and it requires openness and effort to accommodate those of another professional discipline. Even when understood they may still cause problems between professions, and also within professions where these contain different schools of thought. With more than one frame of reference questions arise as to which has the greater validity, and which will prevail. Assessment of a situation made from different viewing-points may result in recommendations for different methods of help. For example, differences may arise between medical and social work practitioners when compulsory admission of the mentally disturbed is under consideration.

The troubles that are commonly presented to a particular profession influence its attitudes to the user. Traditionally doctors, for the benefit of their patients, have had to shoulder responsibilities of life and death and make quick decisions in areas to which the layman could not contribute usefully. Diagnosis is often precise and couched in professional terminology, a specific form of treatment recommended which may require highly specialised knowledge, skills and technical resources. Problems presented to social workers are more often related to ordinary life circumstances arising out of poor personal and social conditions and in many cases there is less reason to make a quick or authoritative decision. Further, a solution which does not take into account the whole situation and actively involve the people concerned is less likely to be lastingly effective. The person with the trouble is usually the primary focus of the doctor; the family or social context may be equally important for the social worker. Their definition of the trouble is framed in everyday language and may be imprecise, except where statutory authority is involved. Even then the view of the situation still includes the family and social context.

It is out of these different conditions that very different attitudes to the user have developed. The term 'patient', which describes the user in relation to the doctor, is defined in the dictionary as: 'A sufferer. One who is under medical treatment. A person or thing that undergoes some action, or to whom or which something is done; a recipient'. The common factor in these definitions is the passive position of the patient. The doctor's complementary modal role is active. The approach to the user which is generally given value in health care is that of an actively benevolent authority figure. For social workers the concept of self-determination is an important value underpinning their attitude to the user. The term 'client' was adopted because, like the client of a solicitor, it defined a more active mode of relationship for the user.

Lack of understanding of these valid differences between practitioners in health and social care can lead to mutual irritation and devaluation of each other's contribution to the helping task. Social workers often find it hard to accept the way in which doctors reach quick and authoritative decisions without involving the user and other people concerned, and without considering its effect on the wider aspects of a person's life and family. Doctors are equally irritated by the slow and equivocal manner in which social workers come to a decision, by the amount of time they spend in helping the person or family to participate in the process of decision-making, or by their open-ended way of working. Following a number of meetings chaired by social workers, a consultant psychiatrist said: 'I know that collaborative processes are slow compared to the way I am used to working but I feel as if, though trained to be a racehorse, I am having to work like a carthorse'.

For a profession to be sufficiently understood by others it is essential that a core professional identity is established even if there may be many variations in its extended identity. The lack of a readily identifiable professional image affects collaboration in that there is no well-established stereotype from which other workers can begin a relationship. Doctors know that their core work is covered by the phrase 'medical care and treatment'. Social workers have not coined an equivalent term to 'treatment', 'casework' no longer serving adequately. Lack of a generally accepted umbrella term covering professional practice makes it all too easy for others to say 'I don't know what they do', and this reflects negatively on the profession's identity. The word 'enablement', is a comprehensive term which covers work with both individuals and families, and describes help that includes a number of non-specific methods frequently used in social work, such as problem-solving, counselling, psychological and material support. It offers a parallel term to treatment and lends itself to the phrase 'social care and enablement'. An adequate professional language is essential in establishing a strong professional identity for practitioners. Equally, an adequate collaborative language is essential in order to establish a strong common identity between faceworkers who need to work together. The individual professional language and the language of collaboration have their place alongside each other.

Insufficient knowledge of other agencies

The following example illustrates how separatism, arising from lack of understanding of another professional's role, can be compounded by lack of knowledge of that worker's agency and its constraints on its workers.

Whose baby?

A mother had arranged for an older child to take her baby to the day nursery because both she and the father had to leave early for work. One morning the nursery head refused to take in the baby, as she thought it was ill. She was unable to contact the mother because the latter had, on changing jobs, failed to give the nursery her new phone number. The nursery head therefore sent the child and baby home, phoned the area social work office and spoke to the family's social worker. The latter went to the home, thought the older child was good with the baby but too young to be left in charge when it was sick, and took them both to the family doctor's surgery which, by this time, was over and the place closed. They then went to the casualty department of the local hospital, where the baby was admitted.

This case was discussed between the paediatrician and social worker in a meeting on collaboration in relation to the under-fives. The paediatrician said that once the baby was in the hospital it became her responsibility to find out what was wrong with it, but she should never have had to do this because the baby was not seriously ill. If she had been working as a GP she would have treated the baby at home. She already had too much work to do. She had spoken to the nursery head who said she had never thought the baby should go to hospital, merely that it should not be in the nursery, because of the danger of infection. The paediatrician criticised the social worker for having brought the baby there, saying that, if she could not reach the GP she should have gone to the health visitor.

With some heat, the social worker said that she also had too much work to do. She had relied on the opinion of the nursery head, who was a nurse, that the baby was ill, so there would have been no point in getting another nurse's opinion. Being unable to contact the GP and already being very late for an important appointment with another client, she had decided that the safest and quickest way of handling the problem was to take the baby to the casualty department of the hospital. She realised now that, when the nursery head had phoned, she should have asked her just how ill the baby was and discussed with her the best thing to do, but this had not occurred to her at the time. The nursery head had been extremely brief and sounded harrassed. All she wanted to do was to unload her responsibility for having sent a sick baby away in the care of a ten-year old girl. Finally, the social worker rounded on the paediatrician: 'You and she have both treated me as if I was the one responsible for the situation. Neither of you seem to have been critical of the mother. After all, it was her baby'. She then pointed out that neither the skills of her profession nor the functions of her agency included the task of physically caring for the sick, though it did include protecting a child at risk.

This example shows a lack of understanding both of the social worker's role and the function of her agency. It is increased by the two other professionals identifying her with the user and turning her into a scapegoat; the social worker, through standing in for the aberrant mother, became her stand-in as the target for criticism. We also see the way in which practitioners are influenced in their attitude to workers in other agencies as a result of identification with their own agency. The nurse, by virtue of being in charge of a nursery, had as a priority the need to get a sick child off the premises whilst making sure that the child was all right. The latter responsibility she passed on to the social worker. If she had been a nurse in a health centre, she would have acted differently. The paediatrician, having been called to the casualty department and finding the home situation unsuitable for a sick baby, felt obliged to admit it and, once in hospital care, to carry out a thorough investigation. Had she been working as a GP she would have made an initial diagnosis and kept the child under supervision. Both worked under pressure and were concerned for the totality of their own work; neither had considered that this was equally true for the social worker.

The working-role of the nurse, doctor and social worker was determined for each of them by their agency and influenced by its current over-stressed situation. Their attitudes, as practitioners, were their own. The social worker's working-identity seems to have lacked strength, and this gave power to the nursery head to define the social worker role for her. Too readily the latter accepted total responsibility for the situation, instead of insisting that the nursery head shared it with her and that together they worked out a sensible plan of action. Both the nursery head and the paediatrician manifested separatist attitudes in their unrealistic expectations of the social worker and her agency, which were reinforced by their narrow agency-orientated viewing-point. Other workers fulfilling the same roles might have reacted differently. If there had been greater collaboration at the initial stage of the problem, the outcome might have been different, and time and money saved.

Again, in the example of referral problems (Chapter 11), had there been better appreciation of the difficulties of the other agency, collaboration might have been easier. In that case however ignorance seemed to be the result of the strong transboundary defences at work. In the present case, rather than a defended outlook, it seemed to be the separatist attitude of a narrow agency viewing-point coupled with ignorance that caused the collaborative problem.

As the situation came up in a discussion group soon after it had occurred, the air was cleared, mutual understanding between paediatrician and social worker established and hangover prevented. Frequently misunderstandings resulting from comparable situations never get discussed between the people concerned or, if they do, not in a place where they can be adequately sorted out. Instead, ignorance and ill-feeling persist, building up an ill-founded image of another profession or agency, as shown in the situation over Bill Bowles' rehousing (Chapter 2).

The agency profile

If agencies are to be fully and appropriately used they must have a well-defined identity which is readily knowable to those who may need to use them. Insufficient information about other agencies is often the cause of collaborative non-events. Modern technology is making it easier but, even if information is available, obtaining the necessary details for deciding on a referral is not always easy.

'Hard' information about an agency – its basic purpose, fields of help, categories of user and trouble served, general methods of help, staffing, the structure of its setting, its referral procedure – can be prepared without too much difficulty. To come by it is often less easy. Information about agencies is usually supplied by the organisations responsible for them, and is published separately by the health service, local authorities and voluntary agencies.

'Soft' information is often difficult to obtain. It covers the agency's helping approach and ethos, the more detailed methods of setting and facework help, length of waiting-list, current priorities and current limitations. Such information may be difficult to formulate, liable to fluctuation, or not for general distribution. However, these are often the factors which determine whether an agency's service is the right one for a particular user.

Agency directories

Two projects were undertaken for compiling directories of the mental health services available to residents in two halves of one borough. Because two district health authorities served the one borough and each served half of a neighbouring borough, the directories were based on the geographical areas served, not on either the borough or the health authority area. The aim was to make them user-friendly by only including information relevant to the particular area. It proved to be extremely difficult to get those at managerial level in the relevant authorities to grasp the rationale of this; each authority assumed that their own catchment area should form the basis of such a directory. To think in terms of a residential community rather than of an organisation required a shift of viewing-point difficult to make. For those who worked at ground level it immediately made sense.

Even when a local directory of services for a particular field of help has been prepared information may not include many of the agencies outside the locality which are able to serve its residents. In each of the directories over 50 relevant agencies were listed. These had mental health (including drug dependency and alcoholism but excluding mental handicap) either as their main purpose, or as a statutory duty in relation to mental disorder. Some of those located outside the area were specialised and might seldom be needed, but none the less could be invaluable for a particular user, for example a drop-in centre for adolescents situated in a neighbouring borough.

The compilers of both directories met with similar problems in their task. The questionnaire was carefully designed so that information could be supplied in a standardised and concise form. Some agencies completed and returned it promptly. It was apparent that they had already put time into shaping the agency-image they wished to present and that this had been agreed by the relevant faceworkers and managers. Others came up against difficulties. First, who was to fill in the form? In large agencies in which mental health was only one of their purposes, was this to be done by those who fulfilled this function or by someone higher up the managerial line? Who was to agree the form, once filled in? – to what managerial levels did it have to go? – to which faceworkers?

Often these issues were ignored in the early stages and it was only when a final proof was sent to the agency for checking that the importance of man-agerial sanction and faceworker backing was realised. At the eleventh hour, agency meetings were held and subtle shifts were embodied in the redrafting. It was clear that many workers felt extremely concerned that the agency image should reflect their own view of it, and there were many different views. Sometimes practitioners in senior positions working independently of each other, such as consultant psychiatrists, had different approaches; sometimes there was a discrepancy between the views of those who shaped agency policy and ground level workers.

It was important to every worker that the best possible image was presented, in order to stand comparison with other agencies. The directory compilers were sometimes faced with lengthy negotiations and difficult decisions, when, from their knowledge of the area, it was evident that an agency's description did not tally with the way it was known to function. In each such case the services included in the description might have been carried out by the agency but because of the constraints under which it was operating or the high prio-rities given to other fields of help only a very limited service was actually being provided. Even though this was well-known in the area, presentation of an unrealistic image still seemed necessary. Practitioners felt it would be a slur on the status of their profession and agency if the mental health work of which they were capable was not included in the directory. Oversell was equally a problem with agencies recently set up; their agency image was as yet not well-established and they saw the directory as an opportunity for promoting it. They either presented the agency as they hoped it would become rather than as it was, or else their description was too vague to be useful.

The difficulties met with in compiling these directories show up various hindrances to ground level collaboration. The agency image which is promoted in a published agency profile is clearly of importance to managers and faceworkers alike. For the latter, because of their identification with the agency, its image affects their own working-identity which, in turn, contributes to their own self-image. This accounts for their need to oversell and for their rivalry with workers in other agencies who seem to have greater opportunity to use their professional skills. If the profile is not printed much can be left vague. At ground level this can lead to a bad agency image, manifested in remarks, such as: 'I don't know what they do;', 'They don't do what they say they do', 'When I phone them, they are off-putting and say they haven't time'. This is likely to leave a bad taste and lead to the agency not being properly used for the tasks which it does perform well.

Where agencies are small, all workers may have a hand in fashioning an agreed agency image. Where local agencies are under the control of a supra-agency, such as a social services department, higher levels of management have final authority. However practitioners still have a subtle influence on the agency image through the way in which they interpret policies or assess cases, and through their special skills and helping approach. Time is well spent when management and faceworkers jointly prepare an agency profile, since they understand better their respective positions and mutual trust is increased. It also facilitates ground level collaboration, because faceworkers become clearer as to the contribution they are empowered to make in any particular case, knowing that they will be backed by their management.

Agencies are not static and directories, even if kept up-to-date, can only serve a limited purpose. Nor can they ever provide all the information necessary for the success of some referrals.

Mrs Rolands, referral confusion

A health visitor had been regularly visiting Mrs Rolands, the mother of a small child. As time went on, Mrs Rolands sought help with her emotional problems, so the health visitor suggested a particular centre which she knew offered long-term therapeutic counselling on a one-to-one basis. The case was handed to a new worker who practised family therapy methods not previously used by the agency. He wrote asking Mr and Mrs Rolands to attend together. Mrs Rolands took the letter to the health visitor, saying that she had not asked for her husband to be involved nor did she wish it. The health visitor was annoyed with the agency and phoned the worker. The latter was annoyed with the health visitor for having made assumptions about the way he worked, but she explained why she had every reason to make these assumptions of his agency.

In presenting this case the counsellor said that he had to agree with the health visitor that if the case had been allocated to another worker it would have been handled as she had anticipated. He realised too late that if he were going to work differently from the way in which the agency was known to work he must first make this clear to the referrer. In the event Mrs Rolands was offered an appointment on her own with a different worker.

This example shows how important it is for workers to be aware of their agency's perceived image and to provide accurate information. It also illustrates the value of sorting out a problem. If the health visitor's irritation with the agency had led her immediately to refer Mrs Rolands elsewhere, the negative hangover might have prevented her making future referrals. The counsellor would have blamed the health visitor and been deprived of feedback from which he would learn something about collaborative practice.

Ignorance of the patterns of practice which result from an agency's primary function is sometimes a cause of difficult interagency relationships, as the following example shows.

Generalist and specialist

A GP was criticised by a social worker for not seeing a case speedily enough that she had considered to be an emergency. He replied that in the past he had been criticised for keeping all his patients waiting because he did not work by appointment. Now he had a system in which he booked two patients every quarter of an hour, and allowed time at the beginning and end of his surgery for patients who came without an appointment. For those who needed longer than seven minutes, unless the trouble was urgent, he made a further appointment outside surgery hours. He had found this worked, although it was always difficult to keep to a timetable. However, it meant that if someone arrived in the middle of a surgery they usually waited till the end. Feeling unwarrantably criticised, he went on to describe some of the difficulties of his job, particularly the great variation in amount of work. When under pressure, he had to balance the needs of one patient against those of others, always making quick decisions. An area social worker said that having heard this she now felt more sympathy for GPs, particularly as when she was the duty officer she was in just the same difficult position. She thought that social workers in agencies whose intake was carefully regulated did not understand the stress of working where there was little possibility of intake control. Based on this common denominator the alliance between GP and area social worker led to a discussion on the kinds of initial assessment that could and should be made according to the function of the agency.

Separatism and role-care

Faceworkers, professions and agencies have a valid interest in maintaining their identity, sphere of functioning, status, authority, funding and scope for development. Each organisation should be concerned to further its own development and take care of its members and the roles they carry. Such *role-care* has four aspects: *role-maintenance* – ensuring that the role is appropriately defined and that the skills and resources are available to fulfil it; *role-development* – increasing skills or enlarging the area of operation; *role-promotion* – enhancing the role's image; and *role-protection* – ensuring that the role is not encroached upon, eroded or devalued. These functions of role-care are essential to good practice, but it is when they cease to serve their primary purpose, that of providing optimum service to the user, and pursue sectional ends that they deteriorate into separatism. Then role-maintenance becomes *status-maintenance*, the harmful effects of which can be seen when the power-position of a profession is used to define the roles of others in such a way that the status of the latter is demeaned in order to enhance that of the former. Role-development deteriorates into *expansionism* at the expense of other workers or agencies. Role-promotion turns into *oversell*. This is often noticeable in developing professions, where the level of competence is inevitably variable between practitioners filling posts of the same grade, and claims for a certain level of competence cannot be substantiated overall.

Role-protection can deteriorate into *protectionism* – the protecting of sectional interests, whether of a faceworker, profession or agency, to the detriment of the overall service to users. When changes are required – whether by employers, or as a result of legislation – which are deemed incompatible with professional and/or agency identity, role-protection may be necessary; but it is difficult for faceworkers to judge when this is, because of their involvement and because, even if new developments are of value in the long run, growing pains are inevitable. If innovative methods are being introduced role-insecurity may cause a worker to adopt the protectionist practice of withdrawing behind established boundaries and restricting participation to stereotyped responses. Protectionism favours maintenance of the status quo and embattled boundaries.

Protective communication

Separatism may cause transboundary difficulties in communication, through the use of a number of common *protective devices*. The case of Mrs Gould (Chapter 2), illustrated the device of *negative consensus*, when views are suppressed and only lip service agreement accorded. Akin is the *hidden agenda*, when the presentation of facts and opinions is designed to lead to a predetermined goal rather than to find the best solution to the user's situation. *Subterfuge* is another such device; faceworkers do not clearly state that they will not undertake certain tasks, but later these are found to be unfulfilled. Overloaded agencies may require their practitioners to be extremely cautious in taking on work. Unless empowered to state openly their agency's priorities in relation to the limited help it is currently able to provide, faceworkers try to avoid accepting work without detracting from the agency image, by subterfuge or a hidden agenda. Such a protective position, even when not clearly recognised, is often sensed by other workers, and leads to an unidentified feeling of frustration.

Practitioners may use these devices on their own behalf as well as their agency's to protect their professional image; for instance with the intention of avoiding taking on a case for which they feel insufficiently skilled. There are some users with mental health problems who 'go the rounds', and seem to be impossible to help adequately. They may be the subject of hidden agendas, in attempts to get some other agency or faceworker to take responsibility for them. If practitioners can openly admit their inability to help effectively, then even if no alternative solution is found for the user's situation at least there will have been a meaningful discussion related to the user's needs and the limitations of skills and services.

Fear of losing face causes workers to maintain a *protective silence* in order not to expose doubtful practice or possible lack of objectivity, so that valuable subjective reactions are sometimes suppressed; or they may resort to *rationalisation* – when specious reasons are given to justify an opinion or an action. For the same reason they may not seek clarification of a point made or a term used which they have not fully understood.

Words themselves may be used protectively. In a discussion about jargon, the process of *mystification* through the use of medical or other technical terms was identified as a means of enhancing the practitioner's self-image or protecting it by hiding the fact that they do not know. Social workers said they wrapped up their uncertainty about how to act with the phrase 'take appropriate action'. The problem does not lie in the particular words, which change with changing fashion, but in the cover-up use to which they are put, the negative effect on others, and the stultification of productive discussion.

The power position

The use of power is not always obvious but is always of relevance to collaboration. It can be used for the benefit of the user or subtly perverted to separatist ends. *Power* is the ability to act or affect something strongly; *authority* is sanctioned power; it may be accorded by common consent, custom or common law. In addition, *practitioner-power* derives from statute law in the form of *statutory powers*, and from delegated authority which gives them *accessing power*.

Practitioners also hold *influential power* which, although not authorised, is appropriately theirs. This comes, first, from professional standing which may be enhanced by its identification with an archetype such as the healer. Second, it comes from the individual practitioner's standing, based on level of competence and the position held in either a professional or agency hierarchy. Third, there is the agency's standing which lends power to its practitioners if they are perceived as identified with a large statutory agency. In a particular case, an agency's function and the degree of its responsibility usually affects the influential power accorded to its representative by those from other agencies, even where statutory authority is not involved; though sometimes power deriving from the profession will override that from the agency. Fourth, self-presentation – the strength and fluency of expression, persuasiveness and conviction. Finally there is the influence of personal standing, a quality recognisable by the respect it evokes in other practitioners. The last two types of influential power can also belong to the user and the carer.

Sapiential power derives from the possession of knowledge that others do not have. This is not confined to the practitioner. It may belong to a technician who is the only person who knows how to operate a complicated machine; or to users and carers, who possess relevant knowledge which they may or may not disclose.

The movement for *empowerment* of users and carers is increasing the awareness of practitioners. Whilst intending to use their power-position for the benefit of users, they may have unwittingly disempowered them, as we saw from the health visitors discussion (Chapter 5). Both users and carers often encourage this by taking the attitude that the professional knows best. Influential power is seldom deliberately used for furthering sectional interests but the discussion on role-definition and on the evaluation of roles in Chapter 9 shows how easily this can be done unwittingly. It requires commitment by practitioners to further a shift in the balance of power, because empowerment of users and carers may well be experienced as their own disempowerment and a threat to their role-identity.

This is equally true of the empowerment of developing professions by those long established. To look at how sectional interests are worked out at national level is not within my province, except to say that it cannot but have a strong influence on secondary collaboration at ground level. Where role boundaries are unclear the situation may be seen as an opportunity for extending the province of the practitioner, in which case there may be competition and rivalry. Alternatively the situation may cause uncertainty-in-role and be experienced as a threat to working-identity; then the overriding need is not to promote identity but to protect it. In either case the worker tries to establish a strong position. Unless the problem is tackled at the appropriate level the result will be continuing rivalry and the introduction of defensive measures.

Overlapping professional boundaries

All the helping professions work in the seven fields of help and the main types of setting. Professional differences lie in their functions, methods, skills and responsibilities, but there are also large *overlap areas* of shared professional province.

Some specific methods of treatment may be carried out equally by doctor or nurse and, in the field of behavioural psychotherapy, by social workers and other professions. In methods of enablement which involve relational skills there is a large overlap. Whilst counselling is a method within the core-province of social work, it also lies within the extended province of all helping professions, as do various types of psychotherapy. There are many facework functions which are shared; for instance, data collection, assessment, opinion and advice-giving, psychological support and network-building. These may be used in a different professional context but the function and necessary skill will be identical and, where practitioners are in the same field of work, some of their work is interchangeable.

An overlap area always constitutes a potential threat to working-identity. This led to the operation of defences in faceworkers in the MIND centre (Chapter 8). In the case of Eddy Edwards, the day centre member (Chapter 2) it caused rivalry which led to protectionist practice, when the preservation of the practitioner's province and status took precedence over the needs of the user.

When relational skills overlap the methods of help being offered may make it clear which practitioner should be carrying out the task, as in the case of Melvin Manson (Chapter 6). Where it is not clear certain guidelines can usually determine who should fulfil the shared method or function. First, *user-preference*: if two practitioners are skilled in, say, counselling, the user may well prefer to talk with one rather than the other. Second, confection of tasks; if a health visitor is visiting a young mother regularly, or a GP seeing a patient frequently for medication, then provided the practitioner is sufficiently competent in relational work the helping-task is likely to be more effective if carried out by a single worker. Sometimes the level of competence is important, as in the case of Mrs Hill (Chapter 3). In this case there was mutual respect between the two practitioners but when this is absent, even though the shared province is recognised, the assessment of relative competence can be hindered by the assumption of protectionist positions.

The existence of an overlap may not be generally accepted by practitioners because they fear that their professional province is being invaded or eroded. And even when the area held in common is clearly defined and the shared province agreed there may still be rivalry for dominance within it.

The terminology which lends itself so readily to describing these collaborative problems shows how closely professional and agency systems resemble ethnic and national systems, and the comparison illuminates collaborative difficulties. Developing professions inevitably create tensions and problems. The following example taken from the early days of the specialism of community psychiatric nursing illustrates the kind of interprofessional problem that arises in relation to levels of competence.

Social workers and CPNs

A team leader in an area social work office had a particular interest in the care of users with mental health problems who lived at home. A newly appointed CPN started working with some of the same users, seeing them for injections at the local health centre, and sometimes visiting them at home and talking with their relatives. This CPN had a natural aptitude but no special training in working with families. His assumption of this role was resented by the social work team leader. She therefore continued to send social workers from her team to visit the same families. The relationship between the CPN and area social workers grew steadily worse. Neither profession would change their way of working. Only when this CPN was sent on a course and his place taken by another who had had some special training in family work, would the team leader begin to negotiate over particular users. Even then, this proved difficult, because the social workers felt their professional province was being eroded. Only gradually could they accept a new area of authentic overlap.

When realignment of professional boundaries is necessary, whether one profession withdraws from a certain sphere of work or remains in it, it is important that the boundaries are clearly redefined and agreement reached on shared province. Whilst this may be possible to plan theoretically, at ground level there is inevitably a difficult period of adjustment during which it is not always easy to distinguish between the restrictive practices of protectionism and the proper protection of the professional province and the user's interests. When innovative methods are not fully accepted by any of the established professions, this will create the same problems. Since needs and services are always changing over time, realignment problems will always exist.

Overlapping agency boundaries

The boundaries of agencies inevitably overlap. If properly defined and managed, these overlap areas can be of benefit in providing optimum help. The primary function of agencies may be identical but if there are variations in their secondary characteristics this provides a range of options to meet users' individual needs. For instance, the provision of day care for those with mental health troubles has a slightly different orientation and ethos when provided in a local authority day centre or a day hospital. The same applies to help from the local community: in the case of Mrs Hill, the depressed single parent (Chapter 3) the different ethos of one playgroup from another was relevant to her being able to make use of such a service.

When an agency is expanded or a new one set up, the working-identity of faceworkers may be threatened because they feel that their agency's status, or even its survival, is threatened. This was evident in the reactions to the opening of a much needed new agency in the field of mental health (Chapter 10). Here the fears were unfounded, but they are sometimes real if a powerful agency with an expansionist tendency does not consult with other agencies before extending its services.

The defended position

Defence mechanisms and separatist processes are to be distinguished from each other by the fact that although both are an automatic response designed to ward off role-insecurity, defence mechanisms operate unconsciously, whereas status-maintenance and protectionism are nearer, if not totally conscious. However they are closely interwoven. For instance, when speaking about an expansion of their own agency workers will see it as providing a new or better service, but when the expansion of another agency is under discussion, the phrase 'empire-building' is not infrequently heard. This may be a true assessment of an agency's separatist expansion, but it may also point to a transboundary defence by which quite natural and not necessarily harmful power-drives are disowned and projected, because of the worker's fear of their own aggressive rivalry.

The following example shows ignorance of an agency which could be the result of a defence mechanism or of separatism.

Referral problems II

When discussing patients with mental health troubles, a GP said: 'I see many whose problems are psychological, but it is not suitable to refer them to a psychiatrist because they are not actually mentally ill, but I am not able to help them myself. The ones who can afford to pay, I send on to a qualified psychotherapist whom I know, but there are some who cannot afford it'. He was unaware that for many years, within a few streets of his surgery, there had been a voluntary agency of high repute, employing experienced social workers who provided a psychotherapeutic counselling service for individuals and families. When told of this agency, he said he had tried to refer to the social worker in the psychiatric department of the local hospital, but had found that the referral could not be made directly and the patient would not wish to be seen by a psychiatrist.

This tangential response seems to indicate that the GP would have found it acceptable to refer to another profession if working within health care or even, perhaps, within the public sector, but that he was not open to referring to another profession in the voluntary sector. He used the boundary of health care, rather than his professional boundary, as a defensive frontier, perhaps because he was employing a defence mechanism which needed to 'down' the voluntary sector in order to 'up' the statutory services; perhaps because of a separatist attitude, which kept him in ignorance of the voluntary sector as a resource.

The following statement shows how a worker with a high level of self-awareness was able to accept her destructive wishes.

A new agency II

In a discussion, a worker from a voluntary agency said: 'When I heard about the borough opening a drop-in centre, my first reaction was very negative. Although we had never put forward the idea, I thought it should have been our agency to do it, and I felt a pang of envy and a wish that it would fail. My next reaction was to castigate myself for being so small-minded, but I did think, and still do, that our agency would have run it better. It is a question for me, now, of how much I shall use it and encourage others to do so'.

She comments on the power she possesses to influence the future of the new project. Avoiding the sour grapes defence, she did not have to shun the project because she had irrationally devalued it. She was then faced with the possibility of adopting a separatist position and, whilst knowing that the project had value, deliberately shunning it. She might then have influenced others to accept her low rating of it as an objectively considered judgement. This worker had a secure role-identity, but the more a faceworker relies for role-security on their professional or agency identification, the greater will be their need to maintain its status, even at the expense of others.

Chapter 13
Province, Domain and Facework Functions:
Collaborative Framework III

In the process of describing common hindrances to collaboration and looking at underlying causes it has become clear that overlapping boundaries can be the cause of difficulty but, when recognised and managed, they can be of great value in the construction of an individually tailored help-compact. Because of the complexity of the overlaps it is useful to have a framework within which to discuss the contributions of professions, agencies and faceworkers to shared tasks. In this chapter I expand on some of the terms I have already used in previous chapters and, with others, order them in a more systematic way.

Professional province

As a working definition, *province* describes the sphere of action of a person or group of people. Within the overall province of helping, each person, including the user, has their own particular province. *Professional province* is based on the fields, settings, methods and functions in which some, if not all, the members of a profession are competent to practise. The province's *external boundaries* will relate to those of users, other professions and groups of helpers, all of whom have their own province. The *sphere of influence* of any group may extend beyond its province. *Internal boundaries* define the smaller provinces, such as branches, specialisms and other subdivisions of the overall professional province. A *branch* of a profession is based on a broad specialisation, often with its own qualifying exams; basic training may sometimes be based on one particular branch of a profession's province, as in psychiatric nursing. A *specialism* is a defined field of help that requires highly specialised professional input; there are many *specialisations* of a lesser degree, which do not warrant the term specialism.

Within a profession, *core-competence* belongs to every member of the profession by virtue of qualification. Practitioners improve their skills, through experience and/or further training, thus acquiring *extended competence*, in any of four *spheres of competence*. *Field-competence* refers to competence in one of the seven fields of help – child care, care of the elderly, physical health, mental health, disablement, disadvantage and social maladjustment. These seven fields can be subdivided into many smaller areas. Child care, for example, includes child health, child abuse, learning disabilities, etc., working in each of which requires some more specialised field-competence. *Setting-competence* refers to the specialised ability needed for working in a particular setting. For example, the routines, procedures and personal comportment required in a hospital will be quite different from those in a drop-in centre. For a practitioner to work effectively in a setting it is necessary to understand something of its organisation and conform to its ways, unless deviating for some valid purpose. Development in *method-competence* and *function-competence* can be through the improvement of core professional skills or the acquisition of new ones belonging to the profession's extended province. In whatever direction they go every practitioner will almost inevitably achieve some degree of specialisation over and above their basic core-competence. It follows that a profession's province is delineated according to the area covered by the core-competence of all, and the extended competence of some, of its members.

Levels of competence, unless there are specific qualifications, have no fixed cut off points but, in a rough threefold classification, practitioners' competence is either *basic*, *proficient*, or *expert* in any sphere of their profession's province. Each practitioner has an individual profile, the two parameters of which are the various levels of competence which they have achieved in the various spheres of competence. This determines the individual professional province or *practitioner-province* – the sphere of action in which they are competent to practise.

To be a *generalist practitioner* in any profession means to be proficient in particular methods necessary in those settings which accept a wide range of troubles and category of user. All good generalists will be proficient in '*first-door' methods* and functions. They are frequently the first practitioner approached by someone with a trouble, and first-door methods are those used in the initial response to a situation. Specialised skills in 'first-door' assessment are needed, to determine: the degree of urgency; the need to contact an existing network; whether to enlist the help of other workers or agencies and, if so, which. The generalist will also have proficiency in certain categories of trouble which do not need the resources of a specialised setting. Generalist practice is as much a specialisation as any other within health or social care.

Internal professional province relates to the branches, specialisms and specialisations within a profession. Some of these are quite distinct from each other, while others have a larger or smaller *province-overlap*. To take examples from child care: the overlap between the specialisms of paediatrics and child psychiatry is large and may cover exactly the same presenting trouble. A child may come into hospital for abdominal pain, the cause of which could be appendicitis or anxiety about going to school. Paediatric and psychiatric competence at a basic level is a component of medical core-competence. Because of the overlap and as a result of working together in the same setting, specialists in paediatrics and child psychiatry may well have acquired proficiency over and above basic competence in the other specialism. Paediatric specialists can rely on their level of competence in child psychiatry or can refer to the specialist, and vice versa. The needs of the user are paramount but, like most guidelines, this is easier to enunciate than to interpret. In the social work profession, the area social worker who is a generalist and the hospital social worker who is working in paediatrics and/or child psychiatry will share core-competence and each have particular specialisations in child care, thus creating their differentiated practitioner-province, but there will be a large province-overlap – similarly with health visitors and paediatric nurses.

The external boundaries of a profession are interrelated with those of other professions. Each has an *exclusive province* which belongs to the one profession only, based on its particular competences, accessing powers and statutory authority; but they all share large areas of province overlap. Because of the overlapping of professional province in respect of spheres and levels of competence it is sometimes possible to reduce the number of practitioners involved in providing comprehensive care. When a generalist practitioner needs the services of another profession at the same time as some specialised input both needs may sometimes be met by one worker. For instance when a GP needs the core competence of a nurse or a social worker at the same time as some specialised field-competence in mental illness over and above the GP's own medical core-competence, they may be able to enlist the help of a CPN or a social worker with psychiatric expertise. Similarly, where a family needs specialised psychiatric help an area social worker may work with a child psychiatrist. In both cases it is important that those involved know when to call in a specialised practitioner of the same profession as the generalist; in the first case, a psychiatrist, in the second, a social worker with special expertise in helping disturbed families.

A subdivision of competence of a different type is based on its origin – from training or from experience – which, as already discussed, can be a source of role-insecurity. Again, as already discussed in relation to developing professions, there can be a wide range of competence found in workers in similar grades and work-roles.

Agency domain

Domain describes the area in which a person or organisation has power to function. As a working definition, an *agency* is a helping organisation which has its own intake system. This description applies equally to a large area social work office and a loosely-structured self-help group, a single-handed GP practice and a large hospital. *Agency-domain* is the area in which it provides a service. This is determined geographically by the *catchment boundary*; and functionally, by the purposes which the agency has been set up to fulfil – *agency-function*. Like individual and professional systems, there are *core* and *extended agency-functions*, the former being fairly permanent, the latter more variable.

Domain-overlaps or *co-domains* are frequent, with innumerable permutations. Whilst providing the same type of setting, agencies may offer different methods of help; or the same methods of help may be offered in either day, in- or out- care settings. Even when very similar, agency profiles are never identical. *Operational domain* is the area of service delivery in which particular help-methods are carried out. When this is contained within the boundaries of a single agency, there is an operational structure, such as a team or a ward, in which operational authority is defined and allocated. When an individual help-compact requires the integration of help-methods from different agencies, there is no pre-existing operational domain. This has to be established through a confederate structure.

Practitioner province and domain

Working-domain is based on the work-role which describes the domain allocated to each worker by the agency. It covers not only a *functional domain* – the tasks they are to fulfil, but also a *discretionary domain* – the area within which they have discretion to make decisions, and a *managerial domain* – the area of responsibility for, and authority over, other workers in a hierarchic structure. A *hierarchy* is 'a body of persons or things ranked in grades, one above another'. A practitioner has a place in two hierarchies, based on professional skill and managerial accountability within an agency, i.e. 'line management'.

Practitioner domain is closely related to practitioner-province since the worker needs a certain competence to fulfil the duties of a particular post. Thus, through the post they hold, practitioners are virtually designated to a particular level of professional competence. However the domain of some practitioners may not include all their professional province, either because of the defined work-role or because the priorities of their agency are such that only certain work can be undertaken.

The *general domain* of a faceworker is defined by their work-role. *Specific domain* refers to the area in which they function in any particular help-compact. If agency boundaries have to be crossed, almost inevitably the domains of the faceworkers will need to be defined in relation to each other: it has to be specifically decided who is going to do what. In routine or simple collaboration, allocation of work-tasks is straightforward. In complex collaboration, the profile of individual faceworkers – their levels of competence in the various fields of competence – and the user's preference will always be important.

When a practitioner has a hierarchic domain, this is implemented through the *supervision* of those accountable to them. Such supervision covers matters belonging to both the worker's domain and province; the two are closely interwoven. The managerial aspect of supervision covers fulfilment of the work-role and the agency's policies – a domain matter. The practice aspect of supervision monitors and helps to improve the worker's professional competence – a province matter. In certain circumstances the two kinds of supervision may be provided by different people – for instance, when the practice of one member of a multi-disciplinary team is supervised by another; or when, in developing professions, training is sought through supervision by a practitioner of another profession.

Where practitioners do not know each other they can only have a stereotype of the others' province and domain, deriving from the professional role and post. An ill-defined professional, agency or work-role image will mean that others have only a vague conception of what can be expected of a particular practitioner. In any event the finer details of a practitioner's domain can never be known except through individual contact, because the personal and competence constituents of working-identity, through influencing the faceworker's interpretation of their role, will affect the content of their domain. The example Whose baby? (Chapter 12), illustrates well how practitioner province is circumscribed by the particular working-domain as defined by their work-role.

The province and domain of other helpers

I have discussed province and domain in terms of practitioners but the concepts apply to all helpers. Each has their competence province – the sphere in which they are capable of functioning, and their *helper-domain* – the area in which they are authorised or have committed themselves to function. The domain of all workers, as with practitioners, is determined by the interpretation of their work-role. Volunteers, however informal the work-role, always need their accountability to be clearly defined as well as having an outline of their duties. This sets limits on what can be expected of them by users, other workers and themselves, and puts controls on what they actually do. The *carer-domain* is based on the commitment the person has given to helping; that of personal carers, on the personal commitment of their relationship and their duties which derive from custom or law. It is further determined by the carer's competence to shoulder responsibility and carry out tasks, and society's attitudes to the provision of back-up help.

The basis of *user-domain* is the human right to self-determination, the duty to respect the rights of others and to look after one's self. This is reduced by lack of competence, from whatever cause. According to the triple aim of helping, the user's normal domain should be maintained as far as possible and the self-helper domain should only be encroached upon for the person's wellbeing.

Facework functions

The carrying of each responsibility and the fulfilment of each constituent task requires a corresponding authority and competence. Because of the large domain-overlap between helpers, including the self-helper, there may be various possible ways of breaking down the overall task into work-tasks. The necessary decisions are facilitated if the faceworkers, particularly practitioners, can define their domain accurately, using a framework and terminology which can be applied to all kinds of practice. For this purpose, I propose the following classification of the skilled functions for carrying out helping-tasks.

- *Investigation/data collection*: through talking, testing and examination, data is collected and investigations made which can throw light on the situation.
- *Assessment/diagnosis/hypothesis*: having collected sufficient data, an evaluation of the situation is made, even if only provisional, to form the basis of a plan or decision for action. Some assessments are made in general terms, some constitute a specific diagnosis, some can only be formulated as a hypothesis which needs further investigation.
- *Opinion/recommendation-giving*: as a result of the foregoing, a view can be offered of the user's situation and the possible ways of bettering it.
- *Information/advice-giving/discussion*: the exchange of facts and perso-nalised views, which will enable plans and decisions to be made.
- *Planning/review*: as a result of the foregoing, a proposal for action is made. Planning may be concerned with a wide range of situations, from help with preparing a weekly budget to considering a major operation or a child's lifetime in care. Often assessment and planning interweave over time.
  - ○ A *plan* defines and programmes objectives, methods, overall helping-task and work-tasks. A plan may be made in outline or in detail. It may be long or short term, firm, provisional or interim, with alternatives, depending on various contingencies. It may be limited to a certain stage of the help-compact, incorporating a review and reassessment at the end of the stage. A review appraises the situation, with possible reassessment and/or changes in the help-compact.
- *Decision-making*: the basis of action to implement a plan or meet a contingency.
- *Authority-use*: the exercise of power to control or influence another person or situation, for the purpose of helping, whether deriving from statutory, professional or personal responsibility.
- *Practical work*: covers every skilled activity which directly produces a tangible result, from that of the home help to the surgeon. Skills vary considerably in their level and range of competence, the degree of spe-cialisation and knowledge required.
- *Relational work*: covers all activity in the area of human relationships,

from befriending to long-term psychotherapy. It includes the establishment and development of working relationships of all kinds.
- *Accessing/referral*: knowing how and having the authority to obtain necessary resources. This includes referral from one agency to another.
- *Compact construction*: combining various elements of helping, through the following.
  ○ *Co-ordination*: the harmonious combination of services to achieve a desired result.
  ○ *Integration*: the making of a whole out of a number of components – a help-compact out of a number of methods.
  ○ *Confection*: an organic process for making a whole by blending ingredients – a work-task out of constituent tasks, an overall helping-task out of a number of work-tasks.
  ○ *Domain-mapping*: defining individual responsibilities and work-tasks in relation to the overall helping-tasks.
  ○ *Communication-mapping*: plotting and setting up the necessary lines of communication for a help-compact.
- *Helper-group organisation/network-building/networking*: setting up the appropriate type of helper-group. This may require: identifying and engaging helpers; defining their tasks, responsibilities and roles; establishing a pattern of working relationships and lines of communication, and ensuring that they function well; organising and chairing meetings.
- *Advocacy*: representing users, where they are unable to present themselves adequately.
- *Monitoring/feedback*: checking on the satisfactory fulfilment of work-tasks and help-compacts. Where necessary, feeding back information to the appropriate place in order to bring about necessary change.
- *Teaching/modelling*: helping users and faceworkers to extend their knowledge and develop their skills through direct teaching or the provision of a model which they can identify with and incorporate.

According to the type of faceworker, their role and their training, these functions will operate very differently. None the less each category has its common denominator. Many of them, even when carried out in quite a different context and concerned with different troubles, require exactly the same skills. For instance the basic skills needed by a doctor and a social worker are identical for helping a user give relevant information, advice-giving, and accessing a service. Relational work is always carried out within a collaborative context and the basic skills are always identical, whatever the professional or agency context.

Domain-mapping and communication-mapping

Domain-mapping defines individual responsibilities and work-tasks in relation to the overall helping-task. It is to facilitate this function that the above framework has been set out. Where the same method of help is frequently provided for a number of users in an identical way, then workers' domains can be mapped on a generalised and long-term basis, though in each case the user's domain will need to be considered individually and those of the workers adjusted accordingly. Priority in domain-mapping goes to establishing the user's domain in relation to the helpers, perhaps to curtail it, perhaps to enlarge it; always seeking the right balance of shared responsibility. Allocation of roles, responsibilities and tasks between practitioners is most efficiently carried out when each one is able to articulate the nature and boundaries of their domain and that of their agency, being clear about the limits of their discretionary domain and the current priorities of their agency.

Unless the task of domain-mapping is specifically allocated it can be initiated by anyone involved in a case. When responsibility for it is in the hands of an operational leader, it can be carried out in an autocratic manner or through consultation with those concerned. When there is no operational leader it can only be achieved by consensus, negotiation or bargaining. However, if the power-position of any helper – more particularly the personal carer or a practitioner – is strong and supported by well-established role-definitions, then that person will have considerable influence in the mapping of domains.

Mapping the domain of personal carers raises two issues: first, whether they have a say in the process or whether their domain is decided for them by the practitioners; secondly, whether it is established more by default than by decision – by what the helping services do not provide. The rights of carers are a political matter, but their needs are a matter of fact. As previously discussed, they often need to be concurrent users and to be supported in their tasks. In long-term home-care, helping the carer and user to map their domains in relation to each other is often an important function of a practitioner. Personally uninvolved, the latter are in a position to weigh up the balance of need between the user and carer, watching as much for over-caring as for lack of care.

The more that informal carers are brought into a situation in which a practitioner has responsibility, the more likely the practitioner is to have a monitoring function as part of their domain. Monitoring is built into the structure of the formal helping agencies but it may need to be specifically mapped in the collaboration between formal and informal carers.

Domain-mapping should always be followed by *communication-mapping*. Lines of communication need to be established so that time is not wasted and each person knows whom to contact and when, the information that is likely to be relevant having been previously clarified. The purpose of communication-mapping is to ensure that people know what they need to know and are not burdened with what they do not need to know.

Where collaboration is complex domain-mapping may be crucial to the outcome of help. Some principles of this function are formulated below:

(1) Whoever is to have responsibility for carrying out a task should be a party, whether personally or through representation, to any decision in which their domain is mapped.

(2) In the domain of decision-making as much responsibility as possible should be carried by the user and then, with safeguards and support, by the personal carer. Good decisions are often the result of discussion and deliberation and it falls within the province of the practitioner to help users and carers to come to a well-considered decision.

(3) Where helper-group organisation is necessary, domain-mapping includes allocation of function-roles, such as co-ordinator or primary faceworker.

(4) Where provinces overlap domains may be decided by: user-preference; the most effective confection of tasks; the particular competence of a certain faceworker; or by negotiation between faceworkers.

(5) Because scarcity of resources may be a factor in domain-mapping, faceworkers may have to use negotiating methods which are more appropriate to planning at managerial levels, such as bargaining.

Domain-mapping and working-identity

The process of domain-mapping, in addition to constructing an effective help-compact, has valuable implications for collaboration. It helps workers to become better informed about the province of professions and the domain of agencies other than their own. Functions which have previously gone undervalued because they have not been clearly defined are highlighted and better appreciated. This applies particularly to tasks carried out by users and informal carers.

Practitioners who are secure in their working-identity will have little problem in mapping their own domain. Those who experience uncertainty-in-role, whether the cause stems from their own position or that of their profession or agency, are likely to find problems in domain-mapping.

Because of the power-position of practitioners it is important that they help users and carers to define their own province – what they are capable of doing – and establish their own domain – what, in the present situation, they are able and have agreed to do. In this way they are helped to become active participants in the allocation of work-tasks. When those in power-positions fully acknowledge the contribution of informal carers, the role-identity of the latter is usually enhanced, with the probable result that they gain greater satisfaction, and often greater competence in fulfilling their tasks.

Domain-mapping concerning relational work is of special importance. Where a person in a power position does not possess a particular skill, they may well minimise its importance or fail to recognise the need for it. Where relational skills are concerned, this will be reinforced if a professional coping pattern based on perceptual fragmentation, withdrawal or the denial of feelings has become institutionalised into a professional defence. When the importance of emotional needs can be recognised by an operational leader who does not possess relational skills then that leader will ensure that, where needed, relational help will form a constituent of the overall helping-task and the domain of a competent worker. The operational leader will also ensure that the user knows that this component of the help-compact is valued. In health care, domains mapped in this way will often necessitate close secondary collaboration; for instance, in the integration of methods for psychosomatic troubles. When users and carers are facing distressing and difficult situations, for instance sudden disability or terminal illness, the confection of relational work with information-giving concerning the prognosis will be of paramount importance, particularly if carried out by different practitioners.

The skill of domain-mapping is essential to all forms of collaboration. The main purpose in setting out this detailed framework is to help faceworkers develop this skill, through raising their level of awareness about what they actually do and how it fits in with what others are doing, and how to communicate this clearly.

Chapter 14
Developing Collaborative Practice

The sole purpose of collaboration, whether primary, secondary or partici-patory is to provide optimum help. The rating of collaborative achievement lies on a continuum, perfect fit at one end and total breakdown at the other; but most is somewhere in between, with a greater or lesser degree of fit or friction. Through good practice some causes of friction can be eliminated or reduced; some seem intractable. Others can act as a stimulus to new thinking, bringing about changes in attitude or developments in practice. In discussing collaborative processes and problems, the attitudes and skills necessary for good practice have become apparent. Here I describe these in a more systematised form. I then discuss ways in which their development can be furthered by professions, agencies and practitioners.

Collaborative attitudes and aptitudes

The troubles presented in a complex situation almost always involve many facets of the user, whether individual or family. I see no helping-approach adequate to such situations except the integrative approach that I have described. Those whose work is fairly circumscribed or who are primarily concerned with highly skilled practical, as distinct from relational, functions need seldom take an active part in complex collaborative cases. For those who do certain clusters of attitudes and aptitudes are desirable, which I group under the terms: reciprocity, flexibility and integrity.

Reciprocity, rooted in respect and concern for the individual, gives value to mutual understanding and the building of mutual trust. It leads to viewing users as potential self-helpers and participants in the helping process. In relation to informal and formal carers it leads to: an exchange of relevant details concerning approach, province and domain; recognition and appreciation of the others' skills and consideration of their feelings; mutual support in fulfilling the overall helping-task; and readiness to work together on transboundary difficulties as they arise.

Flexibility includes readiness to explore new ideas and methods of practice, and an open attitude to change. Subtle relational changes are as important as major developments. For instance: modifying professional character roles and the modal role relationships between practitioners and users and carers; flexibility in defining work-tasks within overlap areas; modifying the relative power-positions of various helpers; modifying agency ethos, particularly concerning the role-definition of users.

Professional integrity puts the user's needs first. Always subscribed to consciously, this can easily be used to provide a cover for furthering the needs of the professionals. Integrity is needed in placing the interests of the whole – whether in the process of domain-mapping, or in the setting up of local projects – above sectional interests. Integrity demands that practitioners examine their own defensive practices and separatist tendencies. Raising the level of awareness of these processes is one of the most important ways of improving collaborative practice.

Collaborative skills

Specialised relational, organising and assessment skills are necessary as a basis for which the practitioner needs to hold concurrently two views of the user, which I term the *dual perspective*. First, the multi-dimensional perspective: perceiving the user as a whole individual in a personal and social context. This view will lead to clearer identification of the user-unit and potential concurrent users, recognition of the need for an integrated help-compact and good use of the resource pool. Second, the linear perspective: being aware of the user's life as a continuous process in time. From this will follow alertness to the root causes of present troubles, appreciation of the work of previous helpers, sensitivity to changing needs with corresponding changes in the help-compact, and recognition of the importance of continuity during any process of significant change, particularly if there is to be a move from one primary faceworker or one setting to another.

Relational skills include: open listening and communicating, and a helping-manner which puts people at their ease. *Open listening* means: hearing, without too much interference from preconceived ideas and judgements; using direction and control for the purpose of hearing more rather than less. It requires the ability to tolerate distress and anxiety without resorting to coping methods that restrict the user's communications, to be alert to the feelings that may be involved in seeking and receiving help, and the effect on people of finding themselves in a user-role with a predefined role relationship, to permit the expression of relevant emotions, and be able to empathise, whilst at the same time retaining the necessary objectivity for fulfilling the helping-task.

Open communication means conveying what seems to be relevant, including feelings as well as facts and opinions, without using defensive methods and protective devices, and expressing this in a form which can be understood and assimilated by those present. Where trust is lacking, defensive processes and protective devices are likely to be operating. It is valuable for practitioners to be alert to them as, even if they cannot be dealt with, recognition of their presence may prevent undue frustration. The need for professional *confidentiality*, withholding certain information about users, may be valid but may also be used as a withdrawal defence. The problem can be reduced if prior to a meeting faceworkers have cleared with users what they are sanctioned to say and to whom.

A *helping manner* manifesting personal concern and professional confidence without superiority enables users, carers and workers to function at their best in a working alliance. The role of carers will not be taken for granted nor undervalued if the practitioner is concerned for their wellbeing as well as that of the user. Whether or not the feeling of being valued results in increased participation it can at least bring emotional benefit to both carer and user.

Over and above these three basic skills there are others which are essential to complex collaboration: *confecting facework functions and work-tasks*, *integrating methods* and *mapping domains* are skills which require understanding of the likely hindrances to good working relationships and ability to resolve or reduce them. When confecting controlling and collaborative relationships with families where protection of the weak is the focus and where authority-use is concerned, the relational aspects of domain-mapping are always important.

Enabling expression of feeling is a skill which can often increase understanding of a situation, resolve blocks to progress, and relieve tension and distress. *Trust-building* is a skill which relies on the practitioner's relational skills but can be greatly increased by an understanding of the need for a secure identity, in user and helper alike.Defensive processes frequently operate in order to avoid feelings of insecurity – if practitioners are aware of this they will be in a better position to appreciate and relate to the underlying anxiety.

Participatory collaboration requires the development of skills in *combining the different role-relationships* of primary and secondary collaboration in the different patterns of a bipartite and group working-alliance. In the more complex situations, the practitioner may need further specialised skills in working with individuals, families and groups.

Organising skills are required to implement the principles of MEC, in: helper-group and network building; domain-mapping; setting up meetings; devising user-friendly referral systems; and managing changes in the help-compact.

Assessment skills in complex situations need to include, whilst retaining the practitioner's own viewing point, a sectional viewing point, and need to appreciate the validity of other viewing points, while recognising that a range of perspectives may be needed to arrive at a satisfactory assessment.

With overlapping agency boundaries, sometimes the problem for the referrer or users themselves is to find the agency most suited to their needs. It is not always possible for a practitioner working in a generalist agency to have sufficient knowledge of the differences between agencies. Specialist agencies in the same field of help will provide a better service if their practitioners make assessments with a view not only to determining whether and how their agency might help, but which agency in the specialised service as a whole would be most suitable for the particular user. Such a practice requires that practitioners have sufficient sense of common identity with the other agencies in their field to know enough about them and to be ready to recommend or refer on to them. Not only does this require added assessment skills, but the absence of a defensive or separatist position.

Professional training in collaborative practice

If it is accepted that the primary collaborative relationship is an essential component of helping, then some training in human relations skills is essential during basic professional training. If it is accepted that the helping approach has a strong influence on practice then students need an opportunity to consider various approaches and reach an individual position.

The essentials of the user–practitioner relationship are similar in all professions. The various helping-approaches are available to members of all professions, though different individuals and professions may start from different basic assumptions. If these two components are seen as common denominators in the basic professional training of all the helping professions, then there is a strong case for interdisciplinary sessions in these subjects at an early stage of training. Since the ability to look at value-systems and the capacity to relate helpfully have little to do with academic ability or specialised practical skills, interdisciplinary training should not present undue problems.

For primary collaboration, practical training is more important than theory in the user–practitioner relationship, through experiential methods of learning, such as role-play, videos and group discussion, and through supervised practice. As well as raising the quality of practitioner–user relationships generally, this would assist those who had little relational ability but much ability in other aspects of helping, to appreciate the value of relational work.

Interdisciplinary discussions on the various helping-approaches would provide a forum in which students, whilst considering their own basic assumptions and evaluating the merits of different approaches, could also appreciate the reasons lying behind differing professional values. If students from various cultural backgrounds were taking part the meaning of a *multi-cultural approach* would be better understood. The process of interdisciplinary group discussion would raise students' level of awareness concerning their professional image and working-identity, the importance of roles to their own sense of identity and their individual methods for achieving role-security. Role-definition considered in an interdisciplinary group would inevitably include that of helpers in relation to users and alert students to the possibility of user-abuse. Such joint training would establish the shared core of practice of all the helping professions, establishing a common identity as faceworkers, beneath professional and personal differences. Solid foundations would be laid for primary and secondary collaboration.

For social workers, proficiency in secondary collaborative practice is a component of their core province and should therefore form part of their basic training. For some health professionals specific training in secondary collaborative practice may not be necessary. For others it is probably better undertaken only after core professional skills and professional identity are well-established. For those who have close contact with other agencies or who specialise in out-care, such as GPs, health visitors and district nurses, post-qualifying training should give them a higher level of competence in secondary and participatory collaboration.

Proficiency in the skills of secondary and participatory collaboration can best be learned through supervised practice and on interdisciplinary and interagency courses and workshops in which a collaborative model is incorporated. If the latter are organised on a local basis and in relation to a specific field of help they have the added value of increasing useful contacts and strengthening mutual trust, thus facilitating local collaboration.

Chairing skills are essential to those involved in complex collaboration who need to set up meetings. Over and above the usual chairing skills and the relational skills outlined above, complex collaboration demands further skills: in deciding whether a case or a participatory meeting or a combination of the two will be most effective in achieving the purpose of the meeting; deciding who should be invited, bearing in mind that the level of professionalism affects the freedom to speak about confidential matters; enabling users, carers and practitioners to relate well enough to each other in a group to say what they need to say.

The contribution of professions to collaborative practice

From the analysis of hindrances to collaboration certain principles concerning professional developments emerge. Professional boundaries need to be clearly defined rather than blurred but, at the same time, shared professional province must be defined and agreed. It is not only in skills and tasks but in responsibilities and authority that changes in professional boundaries are taking place. The implementation of community care policies is causing changes in the relationships of practitioners at ground level and, where there is increased overlap of responsibility, the need for increased collaboration follows.

The fundamental need to protect professional identity and the various ways in which this is attempted have been discussed in previous chapters. It has been shown that temporary coping methods, which are often necessary for efficient practice, can become incorporated into professional practice as permanent defences against role-insecurity. Examples have shown how this can 'damage both primary and secondary collaborative relationships. If this analysis is accepted, it behoves professions to examine their institutionalised methods of handling role-insecurity.

Abandoning defensive patterns is only possible if adequate coping methods are available. It is generally recognised that for individuals the most effective way of alleviating stress is to face its causes, express emotional reactions, and to share and discuss these with someone else. Through this process people are enabled to reach a realistic and stable position in relation to their responsibilities and anxieties and to find realistic and mature ways of meeting the situation. There is no reason why the same should not be true for people when fulfilling a professional role. Given that practice in the helping professions inevitably produces more than average stress, it behoves professions to develop ways to reduce and cope with it. To this end, as well as their specific methods for coping with stress, a profession's image and ethos are important.

Some practitioners with unduly high standards for themselves are burdened by a sense of failure because they cannot live up to their ideal self-image. The result may be overwork, depression, psychological and physical symptoms and the use of strong defence mechanisms. Practitioners are often burdened by identifying with a professional image which, realistically, is beyond attainment, particularly if it is closely linked to an archetypal image to which others may expect them to match up. The same process has trapped women in their mothering role, when they try to live up to the archetypal good mother image. D.W. Winnicott, in helping mothers to escape from the thrall of the unattainable ideal, introduced, in his writings and lectures, the concept of the 'good enough mother'. The 'good enough' concept applied to the professional image would lessen role-insecurity. The 'good enough' practitioner, while accepting that they do not have to be, nor appear to be, perfect, though not content with low standards, can tolerate falling below the ideal. This lessens the need for personal or professional defences; it enables practitioners to acknowledge their failures more easily and, in consequence, learn more from them.

A *professional ethos* which can reduce role-insecurity is one which encourages open communication in the appropriate place and time, allowing stress to be acknowledged and difficulties discussed. Within such an ethos individual practitioners are likely to create their own informal support groups, where they feel secure enough to discard their professional persona, unburden themselves and get help from each other. This may be all that is necessary, but the stress in many jobs may require the coping method of a structured situation, of support, whether set up by the profession or the agency.

If alongside the highest ideals and ethic, such a professional image and ethos can be incorporated into the professional system, it will be internalised by practitioners as acceptable functioning in their professional role. However, the sense of security which is provided by long-established behavioural patterns and institutionalised defences makes change in professional systems very difficult. For this reason, it is of particular importance that desired modifications are introduced and fostered at an early stage of professional training.

The practitioner's contribution to collaborative practice

The following example shows how collaborative practice can be developed and the risk-taking that is involved. The case was presented by an area social worker and a child psychotherapist at an interdisciplinary group.

Mrs Smith: participatory collaboration

An area social worker was offering counselling and support to Mrs Smith, a single-parent mother of a two-year-old daughter. The social worker visited them at home about once a fortnight, talking over problems and giving encouragement. The little girl began to have temper-tantrums which made the mother herself angry and distraught. Unable to help her handle the tantrums, the social worker thought she must seek more expert advice, which was available locally at a children's and parents' centre. She described to the group why it was difficult for her to take this step: 'I felt the centre would be critical of my work and think that area social workers should be able to handle such cases, if they were up to their job. They would then take over the case, and I would feel I had failed'. She thought they would not home visit, and she doubted whether Mrs Smith would attend regularly. She felt the centre workers might be too high-powered, too 'psychological' for Mrs Smith and that she, although unable to help with the tantrums, might understand her better. However, she was worried about Mrs Smith's potential violence. Her senior advised her to discuss the case with the centre's social worker. The latter saw the difficulties in getting Mrs Smith to attend, and suggested that the area social worker should first meet their child psychotherapist. She did so and incidentally saw the centre for the first time.

The therapist then took up the story. Before meeting the area social worker, she had had doubts about taking such a case, wondering whether she would be able to help if the mother was not well enough motivated to come regularly. She felt that with her special expertise she should be able to offer something, but questioned her own ability to do so. When she and the area social worker met, she was tempted to say that the case was not suitable for the centre, thus fulfilling the agency's perceived image, as only accepting the 'cream' of the cases needing help with children's problems. Instead, she decided to share her doubts about her capacity to help. Encouraged by this the social worker shared her anxieties about the superior nature of the workers at the centre. Fellow-feeling emerged and a working alliance was established. The therapist felt she would be better able to help if the mother and child would come to the centre, but that the social worker should come too, remaining the only social worker in the case. They agreed that in the first session they would work on the problem together as a foursome.

The social worker described the next step. Feeling trust in the therapist, knowing what the centre looked like and being clear what would happen when they got there, she found it easy to put the idea over to Mrs Smith in a positive way. She phoned the therapist, agreed a date for the appointment, and the therapist said she would write to Mrs Smith.

The therapist then told how, two days before the appointment, the social worker phoned to say that Mrs Smith had not received the letter. The therapist was horrified to realise she had forgotten to write it. She said that this oversight brought home to her just how anxious she felt at the idea of working in a different way from her usual practice.

In the first session, the therapist played with the child and talked with the mother, discussing toddler behaviour and the aggressive feelings in both of them. At the end of the session, the therapist felt able to reassure Mrs Smith that there was nothing abnormal in the little girl and that many mothers found this a difficult phase of development. They had another session the following week, at the end of which it was agreed that the social worker would continue visiting Mrs Smith at home, and that the therapist would see them in six months' time or at any time before then should they request it. Mrs Smith said she felt much better about the problem and reassured that she could come back at any time.

Here we see a help-compact tailored to the needs of the particular user, the capacities of the particular practitioners and the specific functions of their agencies. It fulfilled the requirements of MEC and, in achieving immediate goals, it was time-efficient. It is impossible to evaluate its long-term effects but these could be considerable, in terms of both human wellbeing and cost-effectiveness. Such a help-compact was only possible because the face-workers, supported by their professional ethic, did not fall into the defensive trap. Instead, they faced the insecurity of not feeling good enough in the shared province where their relational skills overlapped. Their respective reactions highlighted the professional and agency defences which could have been adopted and which would have led, on the one hand, to not making the referral, on the other to not accepting it. Through tolerating role-insecurity the practitioners were able to explore new ways of working and to involve the user as a self-helper in a tripartite working alliance. They were supported by their two senior social workers, whose flexibility facilitated the referral process. At the time, both agencies were attempting to develop new ways of maximising help.

The contribution of agencies to collaborative practice

If agency management is concerned to foster ground-level collaboration, it must provide a firm working-base for its faceworkers. This requires a well-defined and realistic agency profile, which allows the constraints under which it is working to be known by other agencies; good communication between management and faceworkers; well-defined working-roles and adequate support, so that role-insecurity is reduced to a minimum.

To achieve the latter agencies must provide adequate managerial and practice supervision and methods for coping with stress. These needs may be met through various structures such as individual or group supervision, staff groups, operational team meetings, whether single or multidisciplinary. It may be necessary to set up structures with the primary function of coping with stress. To fulfil their objective and be time-efficient, the person in charge must have adequate relational skills. The primary task here is to alleviate stress at work and although stress arising from other causes should be acknowledged and its working out not totally barred, it cannot be a continuing primary focus. A similar principle applies to feelings about colleagues; when connected with specific working situations they are relevant but other feelings, whilst being recognised, have little place in discussion. Boundaries must be clearly drawn and firmly maintained.

Collaborative practice is likely to demand some modification of workers' attitudes, as well as the development of new skills. The availability of groups in which reactions to change and developments in practice can be discussed can reduce the need to retreat into defensive and protectionist positions. If such groups are to fulfil their task it is essential that some members are able to detect and point out the use of group defences. Otherwise discussion may be limited through the projection of inadequacy or displacement of hostile feelings outside the group boundary. At times, it may be cost-effective for agencies to employ social consultants on short contracts, to enable workers to understand more about group relations and to develop effective ways of working together. Voluntary agencies may find it cost-effective to employ a consultant to support their principal worker by providing a place in which that person can deal with stress and clarify their functions and priorities for developing the agency's activities.

Essential to a strong working-base is good communication across hierarchic boundaries. Like other boundaries, these can provide fertile ground for defensive processes to develop. It is necessary to build mutual trust through open communication and the discussion of difficulties. Where rivalry is concerned, just as in interagency situations, clear definition of roles and boundaries can help to reduce and contain it. Within an agency every stratum in a hierarchy except the top and the bottom is sandwiched between two others, with interfaces looking upwards and downwards. At the bottom, the faceworker's downward interface is with the user; at the top, the director or principal worker has an upward interface with an executive committee or other body. Workers need to maintain the distinct role-identity of their hierarchic stratum in the face of the pulls and pushes coming from above and below. It is easy for faceworkers to become over-identified with users, feeling that those above them do not understand their problems properly or meet them adequately; alternatively, if over-identifying up the line, faceworkers may become too bureaucratic and lack an individualised response to the user's situation.

Unless there is open communication it is difficult for faceworkers to appreciate the position of those above them, particularly the latter's need to exercise sufficient authority to ensure fulfilment of their own responsibilities. Workers with hierarchic responsibilities may fear that they will not know what is going on and may lose control over those who are accountable to them; that the latter will not fulfil agency policies and priorities adequately or will misrepresent the agency image. Those below may feel that managers are 'breathing down their neck', allowing them insufficient discretionary power or space in which to develop their individual ways of practising. Alternatively, they may feel inadequately supported, insufficiently briefed about agency policy or unable to count on their management fulfilling its declared policy and priorities and backing decisions which the faceworker has made on its behalf.

Adequate communication down the line is particularly important in large agencies. An inherent difficulty for the practitioner at ground level is that of representation on local committees or working groups. For instance, on an interagency committee concerned with a particular category of user some-one of managerial level will represent their agency, whereas the representatives of small voluntary and informal agencies are likely also to be working at ground level. When in conversation with the latter, agency practitioners may find that less qualified faceworkers from other agencies know more about their agency's policy on certain matters than they do themselves.

In yet another way agency management exerts an important influence on collaboration at ground level. A relational pattern operating at the interface of hierarchic boundaries may easily be transferred down the line to become incorporated as a model for those relationships between faceworker and user which are concerned with the definition of responsibilities and tasks, boundary-setting, monitoring and the use of authority. Where the agency's hierarchic relationships are confused or authoritarian it will be more difficult for faceworkers to work collaboratively at ground level. Conversely, where collaborative attitudes and skills are incorporated in hierarchic relationships, the model will facilitate ground level collaboration.

It is essential that agencies, departments within agencies, or teams encourage the working out of internal problems. Otherwise defensive processes become necessary and internal harmony is likely to be maintained at the expense of external relationships. Good internal relations are furthered by an agency ethos which encourages openness and free discussion, within the constraints of time-efficiency rather than the constraints of defensiveness. If the ethos incorporates human values, such as concern for the wellbeing of fellow workers, respect for individuals regardless of position, and recognition of their contribution to fulfilling the agency's functions, it is likely to create an atmosphere in which workers feel they have a valued place. A sense of belonging and of personal value encourages group cohesion and strengthens commitment to the agency's aims.

Collaborative infrastructure and the faceworker

Ground-level structure is important in facilitating transboundary collaboration. The organisational structures and guidelines already developed for categories of user where statutory authority is involved offer models for collaboration in specific situations in which managerial responsibility is involved and where there may be a case for the establishment of specialised liaison posts. Here I look at the development of a more generalised collaborative infrastructure.

Many faceworkers contribute to building an infrastructure, through individual working relationships and informal network groups. If an integrative approach is to be fostered the collaborative infrastructure needs to be related to a particular locality. Then the infrastructure would bring together the faceworkers who serve it, regardless of their agency's total catchment area or geographical position, helping to develop a shared identity in serving a particular group of people.

In developing a local infrastructure specific initiatives are likely to be of value, such as: preparation of computerised local directories; development of general networks for specific fields of help and liaison groups between workers in agencies with closely interlocking functions; a focus on user-friendly referral systems and on finding solutions to the problem of contacting other workers at convenient times; provision of local interdisciplinary and interagency workshops, related to a particular field of help or particular relational skills.

There is a danger that faceworkers spend increasing time away from direct contact with users with no tangible results to show for it. Collaborative work is often a vaguely defined part of the working-role without any specific priority and when individual workers put effort into it the value is not always maximised, because the contacts are uncoordinated. On grounds of time-efficiency there is a case, in certain agencies, for designating a specific function-role of *local collaborator* as part of a practitioner's work-role, allotting it priority for a given amount of time. Unless specific time is sanctioned, it will take low priority. Combining the role with a facework role would ensure that it was not detached from ground-level work. This would enable local collaborative developments to spring from the grassroots and be closely related to the local community and its needs.

The work would focus on developing and maintaining the agency's collaborative relationships at ground level, co-ordinating its faceworkers' contacts into a clearly defined agency network. It is not the links with the various resources that need to be in the hands of one person but the overview. Each faceworker should be clear what information they need about local services; the local collaborator would see that this was available and would ensure that contact was maintained with relevant workers and that time was not spent on unnecessary contacts.

There is a need for establishing a system for feedback concerning collaborative difficulties at grassroots level so that they can be resolved or at least better understood. A local collaborator with special skills in transboundary relationships could advise and help colleagues sort out transboundary problems as they arose, the aim being to minimise the hangover of bad feeling, maximise the possibility of learning from experience and identify areas where change seemed necessary. In addition, the role might include contributing to any of the initiatives listed above.

Future developments

I have outlined above some suggestions for developing collaborative practice; not a massive list but requiring considerable motivation to implement, as they involve changes in attitude and in long-established patterns of professional and agency viewing-points and institutionalised defences.

These suggestions stem from an integrative approach based on a model of the helping scene in which each agency and potential source of help is viewed not only as an independent unit but also as a subsystem of an overall helping system. If this is to become a reality rather than a model, a shared identity will need to develop amongst faceworkers serving a local community, in addition to their agency, and professional identifications. A shared identity and common objectives help to overcome defences and separatism, into which practitioners can easily withdraw during periods of large-scale change.

It is not within my province to comment on reorganisation in the helping services, except to make three points. First, that during such a process the provision of methods for coping with stress are particularly important. Second, that however much relationships between agencies are restructured and however many interdisciplinary projects are set up the problems of working across group boundaries do not disappear. Third, that the hindrances to collaboration which have been discussed here in relation to transboundary relationships between faceworkers can also operate at the boundary between practitioners and managers. If the helping services are to meet the needs of users in their local community, then a relational approach to developing collaborative practice across this boundary is as important as it is at the point of delivery.

Chapter 15
Working Together: Towards a Collaborative Ethos

I come back to the first example I gave, in Chapter 1, which was taken for a discussion on a course organised by an NHS centre for psychotherapy, and now follow the discussion to its conclusion.

The opening scene concluded

A group of about 30 practitioners from various professions and agencies in a particular inner-city locality are discussing the difficulties of helping disorganised families with multiple problems.

TEACHER: As I've said before, when the parents of my pupils are being helped by other people, I find it odd that so often they don't make contact with me. Why don't they?

HEALTH VISITOR: When you speak about 'my pupils and their parents', I keep on thinking 'these are my families'.

SOCIAL WORKER: But they are my clients.

GP: (half joking, but with feeling) Not to be outdone, I must establish that they are my patients.

AREA SOCIAL WORKER: I get angry with hospital social workers who speak about 'my patients' when they are talking with doctors. Why don't they say 'my clients'? After all they are social workers.

HOSPITAL SOCIAL WORKER: Sometimes I feel I'm more in tune with doctors than I am with area social workers.

TEACHER: We were discussing disorganised families not disorganised social workers! What I wanted to know, was who should take responsibility for contacting other workers.

The discussion came back to the families with problems and the responsibilities of practitioners. Some criticism was directed at social workers in the local area office.

AREA SOCIAL WORKER: We don't always get the support we could wish, particularly from GPs.

HEALTH VISITOR: You can't get out of it blaming someone else.

SOCIAL WORKER: (angrily) Well health visitors can visit and be seen as kind and helpful, and the social workers get turned into the 'baddies' because they have the power to take children away. You hide behind us.

ANOTHER SOCIAL WORKER: Often in this group you have been hinting that we were not doing our job properly. You seem to think you know it all.

It was true that this health visitor had taken a didactic attitude.

HEALTH VISITOR: (after a short pause, and in an unexpectedly distressed voice) I don't know it all. I wish I did. Sometimes I feel I am no help at all to the families I work with.

(silence)

SOCIAL WORKER: I feel just the same.

A wave of fellow-feeling swept the group. The tone changed completely. Suddenly people were free to express doubts about their work. They spoke of cases which had gone from bad to worse or certainly had shown no signs of improvement.

SOMEONE: Sometimes I go home at the end of the day wondering why I do this job. It all seems so hopeless.

ANOTHER: There are so many problems that are beyond us to put right.

(long silence)

HEALTH VISITOR (who had sparked off the discussion): I feel better having said what I did, because I realise that I'm not the only one, and I do know that sometimes I can make a difference to a family.

SOCIAL WORKER: I know you can, from some of the cases of yours that have come my way.

SOMEONE: Then perhaps we should look at what it is possible for us to do – given that we work in an inner-city area and we're none of us superhuman.

ANOTHER: And perhaps we should see what we can learn from them here.

ONE OF THE CENTRE WORKERS: I wonder if you had the idea that we at the centre were setting ourselves up and thought we 'knew it all'.

(laughter)

I gave the first part of this exchange in my first chapter, because it was in group discussions like this that I began to see some of the subtle hindrances to collaboration. Many of the participants in these groups knew each other already, sharing cases and referring to each other's agencies. This was an unusual feature for a course of this kind. However, the fear that it might inhibit free discussion proved groundless. Instead, an unforeseen dimension was added: the issue of collaboration between workers in agencies serving the same locality.

Particularly in the large group, participants felt isolated and had a need to establish some shared identity. In the meeting described above subgroups are seen to emerge, first based on professional identification and then, in the exchange between the area and hospital social workers, on agency-identification. The need to establish a shared identity was followed by the need to give it a satisfactory image, and it was perhaps this that contributed to the hospital social workers aligning themselves with doctors in their agency. In a group of practitioners and other helpers facing inner-city problems the potential sense of inadequacy is likely to be great, and the wish to find a way to defend against experiencing its defeating and depressing effect correspondingly strong. Discussion of the needs of disorganised families touched off considerable uncertainty-in-role and to deal with the feelings of inadequacy two defences were brought into action: the omnipotent defence and the downing defence. The former was indicated through the remark about the health visitor 'knowing it all' and the laughter which greeted the final remark about the centre workers. In using the downing defence, the peg on which to hang the projected inadequacy was not difficult to find, since no profession has an answer to the problems of people living in inner-city areas. The maladaptive function of these defences is clearly seen in that it rendered collaborative relationships impossible.

The session shows the process by which participants developed a response better adapted to the situation. Because the group was able to stay with the feeling of defeat expressed by one of its members, sharing rather than denying it, defensive positions were no longer necessary. Once these were abandoned, workers who a few minutes before had been at loggerheads were able to share reactions to their work, in particular, a sense of powerlessness in front of vast problems. Out of this, positive attitudes emerged, realistically limited and orientated to professional tasks, mutually supportive towards each other, and more open to learning from the course. A more detailed study of the same process was given in the 'Referral problems' (Chapter 11) between two social work agencies.

We see that the negative motivation – the need to defend identity – overlay positive motivation – the wish to improve skills and to collaborate for the sake of those who needed help. To be effective in one's job and to help others are two strong personal needs which seek satisfaction through the helping professions. Identification with the image of an effective helper can be crucial to maintaining a good-enough self-image. Thus, at all costs, the professional image must be protected. It was only when the feared calamity of being identified with total uselessness was faced, rendering redundant the omnipotent and downing defences, that the shared aim could manifest itself in a shared identity; that of the inner-city faceworker up against incredible odds.

A minimally structured large group is unsuitable for achieving tasks or coming to a decision, but it has great value as a means through which to understand the human tensions that can operate below the surface of structured meetings. It also has parallels with the relatively unstructured situations in which practitioners often find themselves when working across agency boundaries. The trust that had been built up during the preceding meetings allowed feelings of inadequacy to come to the surface, making working-identity very vulnerable. The above exchange shows the defensive processes operating in an undisguised form; usually their expression is covert, politely phrased in professional language.

At the beginning of the book, the 'Opening scene' presented some of the commonest hindrances to collaboration. Here, at the end, the 'Scene's conclusion' shows what is needed for their resolution. The intervening chapters will, I hope, have enabled the reader to understand more about the many problems of collaboration across personal, professional and agency boundaries. The examples given have been taken from my own field of work but the processes described are relevant to all helping relationships. Focus has often been on practitioners because their collaboration is so important in complex situations and, to achieve it, their special problems have to be addressed. However, helping relationships are not confined to the professionals and the model which I have proposed for an integrative approach gives personal and non-professional carers a valued place, and the self-helper a central position. This provides the foundation for developing a collaborative ethos which would encourage and enable all helpers to make their maximum contribution through working together.

Underlying all the relational problems, for faceworkers and users alike, is the fundamental human need for a secure and satisfying identity, which so easily gives rise to defensive and separatist positions and restricts ability to adapt to necessary change. Although professions and agencies can help in developing a collaborative ethos, in the end it comes back to each individual and their capacity to take risks with their self-image.

Part III
Organisations and Contexts

Introduction

In the previous sections of this book Sally Hornby identified hindrances to collaboration and then suggested ways in which these hindrances could be resolved. The previous chapters will have enabled readers to appreciate the many problems and successes of collaboration across personal, professional and agency boundaries. The focus has been on ground-level practitioners, the 'faceworkers' in any field or speciality who work at the interface with users and carers. Throughout the work the centrality of the self-helper and the nature of helping relationships is maintained since it is so essential for successful collaborative practice. An integrated approach is recommended not least because of the need for uniformity of power relations, maintenance of the value placed on personal and local carers and the need to continuously develop a collaborative ethos in humane institutions and services.

In this section these ideas are considered in the wider contexts of policy making and organisational contexts. Despite many studies on the subject in recent years many people in the helping services are increasingly aware that the level of collaboration achieved between individuals, agencies and professions remains inadequate and often fails to provide optimum levels of care (Finlay 2000). It is also evident that collaboration between helpers and between agencies is still not easy to achieve, not least because collaboration is essentially a *human* relationship rather than one that can be imposed by the norms and structures of organisations.

> "The difficulty is that whilst it takes thirty seconds or so to say 'and there shall be co-ordination between the various forms of provision', the actual, day-to-day carrying-out of this co-ordination is a different kettle of fish . . . behind an apparently rational statement is the whole range of human intractability, incompetence, power politics, greed and negativity, together with, of course, sweet reasonableness, great imagination, creativity, generosity and altruism".
>
> (Gillett, 1995, p. 356)

In terms of collaborative care the humanness of the endeavour can be explained further, not least by the difficulties of working across organisational boundaries and across various contexts of care. At the organisational or structural level the complexities and difficulties of working across the boundaries of different domains, in terms of authorities, specialities, teams and cultures, currently appear to be too strong for many individuals, agencies and institutions. As a result they have begun increasingly to defend their own identities, integrity and, in particular, their resource pools.

Explanations for defensive behaviours in individuals and groups have been explored in the two previous sections. The search for explanations is continued in this section with a particular emphasis on the possible impacts of defensive organisational behaviours on group and team dynamics and the processes and outcomes in terms of effective collaborative practice. The focus is on the need for faceworkers engaged in primary, secondary and participatory collaboration, both individually and in teams, to continue to be able to maintain helping relationships in the face of organisational change.

In Chapter 16 the authors consider possible effects of organisational-level anxiety on the quality of care delivered at ground level. Current case studies are used to illustrate interpretations and perspectives of the nature and quality of ground level practices. These are linked to instances of poor dialogue between ground-level faceworkers and managerial decision-takers, the effects of non-collaborative working, and the effects of successful group learning on local practice. The latter can be seen to contribute both to improvements in the quality of care and to the quality of role-satisfying relationships between faceworkers and clients.

Explanations for current levels of institutional anxiety have been sought from the literature on the psycho-dynamics of organisations, recent government policy initiatives and research studies. Attention is drawn to the effects of failing to address damagingly high levels of anxiety and the failure to prevent any dysfunctional organisational learning that can defeat its own purposes.

Recent case studies and anecdotal examples are again used in Chapter 17 to illustrate how individuals and groups act to enhance or evade procedures, guidelines and legal precedents in order to maintain valued, helping relationships. Analysis and explanations of these behaviours are offered in terms of individual and group motivational learning, reductions in defensive behaviours, and changes to an outward, client-centred approach to the allocation of resources and role-satisfying behaviours among faceworkers.

Chapter 18 provides some recommendations for sharing good practice based on a particular case study. Each of the collaborative frameworks identified by Sally Hornby is revisited with a focus on the organisational contexts. Arguments are presented for addressing issues associated with rising levels of institutional, group, and individual anxiety in the interests of all parties being better able to deal with their own difficulties and improve services for carers and users. Links are established between the themes of Parts 1 – III across the book and conclusions drawn about the implications of relating current policy directives to ground level practices.

Throughout this third section the contributors have striven to maintain the flavour and content of the first two sections in the interest of preparing a cohesive text based on reflective, psychodynamic practice. While the first person, reflective stance taken by Sally Hornby could not be duplicated the contributors have used a very similar approach, identifying themes and issues from the case studies and recent experiences in the contributors' own practices. Shared learning across the team, originally under the leadership of Sally Hornby, has led to new and current perspectives on the nature of anxiety-driven practices and ways of helping to overcome negative consequences and achieve ground level faceworker-client relationships that are satisfying, effective and collaborative.

Chapter 16
Consequences of Institutional Anxiety

Introduction

In this chapter the authors have drawn together a number of factors with regard to some of the consequences of institutional anxiety, notably defensive behaviours and constraints on the achievements of faceworkers in maintaining helping relationships.

The notion of projection is used to illustrate how individuals and groups, overwhelmed by work at ground level which is intensified by the stress of working collaboratively with others and by the inclusion of users and carers into team decision-making, can experience feelings of guilt and failure which are then 'blamed' on managers or representatives of the organisation. A case study is used to generate questions about possible projections and the risk of teams expending energy on self-absorption and concern about the control of professionals by the organisations and groups to which they belong.

The results of group and organisational learning are illustrated by the outcomes of the case study. The threats that change poses to individuals and groups are explored in terms of how team members managed these aspects in positive and collaborative ways, overcoming possible negative reactions in order to achieve shared visions of care and build creative partnerships with users and carers.

The motivational rewards of achievements such as those illustrated in the case study are interpreted in terms of wider organisational learning. However there could be a failure to learn as a result of the tendency of humane organisations to be overly ambitious in defining their tasks and objectives without reference to available resources. These issues are discussed in the context of possible underestimation of problems coupled with inadequate means.

The gap between policy makers at the managerial level in hospitals, NHS Trusts/Consortia or Social Service Departments, and faceworkers at ground level practice, with the concomitant failure to engage in meaningful dialogue, appears to be widening with no relief from recent government directives and consultation documents. It is suggested that the continuation of rhetoric, overly ambitious stated aims and a failure to address the provision of resources contributes to dysfunctional organisational learning, higher levels of angry and disenchanted users, and the potential for a demoralised and disenchanted workforce.

The fight for resources

There is evidence that defensive organisational behaviours can have a direct impact on the quality of interprofessional relationships and on multiprofessional practice at the faceworker/user interface. This can result in the alienation of some users and a considerable waste of resources (Lucas et al 1997). Defensive behaviours, possibly due to managerial anxieties, can lead to dysfunctional organisational learning. This can lead to a failure to adapt adequately to changes in the demands and constraints arising from political and social changes in the environment of the organisation (Buckley, 1981).

However, Khaleelee and Miller (1993) suggest that attributions of blame for uncomfortable feelings from those within the organisation can be seen as negative projections onto some sort of faceless 'them'; the hierarchy, or the 'system'. In terms of health and social care such psychological projections may be a particularly prevalent phenomena at times when there is an increase in the size and complexity of ground level work beyond the known and familiar patterns of practice, and these factors cause an increase in stress levels. Projection as an attempt to remove a sense of failure from oneself onto those higher up in the organisation can act as a defensive mechanism, leading to an expression of desire for a redirection of attention towards what is needed for a more successful system. The authors' experiences show that a trigger such as a complaint may be needed to break the cycle of negative projections and induce a review of perceptions and practices.

The following example comes from a focus group discussion with members of a carers' forum in December 1999, on the subject of their experiences of multiprofessional practice. The case may help to make a distinction between anxiety at the institutional level and projections into the organisational level by users and faceworkers.

Focus Group Discussion

Carer:

In my view miscommunication arises from management who do not seem to know what happens at the coalface. Everyone is fighting for their bit of money and (because of this) communication breaks down completely and this puts pressure on professionals all the time. Often it is a complaint that brings all this to the surface like when the Nutrition Project was set up in the Community Hospital. Someone complained about their relative being very hungry and a study was set up. It came out that 40% of the patients in the hospital were malnourished often because patients could not physically feed themselves. The professionals were all so busy and pressured that they had not communicated with the patients or the helpers who gave out the food. So it was not wilful neglect but they are required to do so many things that they can't manage. People can't get better if they do not get nourishment.

I heard from Mr Brown at our AGM how he had written down everything about his wife who was admitted, including about her food, but then found that his notes had been totally ignored and not passed on. When she had not eaten her food the staff thought that she was not hungry and took it away. In fact she could not reach the tray and could not speak to say what she needed because she had had a stroke.

The extract indicates the way in which this particular carer interpreted the situation and concluded that the results of pressures on staff, from the point of delivery of services, arose from too many demands by the managers in the organisation. Such a projection of their interpretations caused them to express considerable degrees of anger and some amazement at the lack of common sense and decency from a service that supposedly worked to high standards of effective care. However, it is noteworthy that the carers projected blame onto the managers for the pressures on the staff, and interpreted managerial inadequacy as the cause of poor inter-staff communication.

There were obvious contradictions closer to home, such as normal expectations of professional staff who should be able to meet the basic needs of the users and to communicate with each other about the details of required care. However these were apparently ignored by the carer in favour of defending the professionals, whom the carer saw as working excessively hard in the situation. It appears that the carer suggested that the situation was to some extent excusable at the ground level, since they perceived that the work was complex, rushed and did not offer opportunities for careful assessments of the care needs of individual users. The carer appears to mean that the opinions of the faceworkers, and indeed of the users themselves, are seldom heard. The carer perceived limited or non-existent opportunities for either informal open discussions, or more formal means of detecting changes in the complex operational interface between the faceworkers and users. The carer saw the need for communication of these problems – heavy workloads and the pressures of helping an increasing number of people in hospitals – to policy-makers and decision-takers at the managerial level of the organisation, if the level of care was going to improve.

As has been described throughout this book the nature of the carer/user interface with faceworkers at the ground level is intensely psychodynamic; it is built on trust, respect and careful attempts to ensure non-dependent relationships. In terms of collaborative, multiprofessional practice these relationships can be complicated by the constantly changing nature of the trans-boundary transactions between professionals that supposedly contribute to participative teamwork at the ground level. However, ground level practice can be increased in size and complexity by an expectation that faceworkers will work across boundaries of professional identities in multiprofessional practice. These expectations arise from the currently changing nature of health and social care organisations. Furthermore, boundaries of decision-making roles within the hierarchy of health and social care organisations have become more formal and distant. This can lead to less autonomy and less upward communication from the faceworkers and increase the potential for failure to attend to the most obvious immediate needs of the users.

The complexity of ground level practice

A number of possible explanations for the interpretations of the situation can be drawn from the extract, based on notions of psychodynamic factors such as relationship building. One is whether attending to the increasing size and complexity of multiprofessional, collaborative practice moved faceworkers beyond what had been established, in terms of relationships with users, into a need for the reworking of relationships with a variety of professionals. Such a change would be equivalent to moving from what was known and familiar into areas of uncertainty. In such situations faceworkers might be tempted to defend themselves from the anxieties associated with uncertainty by projecting blame for the generation of situations like these, and for their resultant feelings, onto representatives of the organisation. Another explanation is that attending to the needs of the multiprofessional team, in order to sustain team cohesiveness, resulted in a loss of attention to the overall purpose of teamworking. A third explanation is the additional complexity in relationship-building that can arise when users and carers are incorporated into the team.

If the size and complexity of work at the ground level did move the faceworkers beyond the known and familiar patterns of working the situation could have triggered feelings of guilt and failure. It is these features of the situation that could have led the faceworkers to project feelings of guilt about their own lack of confidence and competence towards the organisational goals and policies, since faceworkers often feel overwhelmed by unattainable institutional expectations and requirements.

Collaborative teams can work towards a co-ordinated division of labour and provide holistic, integrated care. However, attending to the needs of the team for sustainable cohesiveness can lead to team members becoming self-absorbed and unduly focused on team relationships, putting these ahead of the needs of users (Finlay, 2000).

The inclusion of users and carers into the team is seen by some as essential if various forms of organisational control are to be avoided (Teram, 1997). Humane institutions have the ability to control both professionals and clients. They can constrain the exercise of professional discretion by making team members subordinate to one professional group or to the culture generated by the team. The presentation of a united front to the user can be intimidating and even punishing if multiprofessional work provides opportunities for pooling control mechanisms. Teram (1997) also raises questions about the appropriateness of negotiations between professionals directly responsible for the care of users and those who are not. Faceworkers can, for example, experience interference from institutional managers if the managers are concerned about the resource implications of meeting complex demands of users in some social or health care situations.

Defensive behaviours

Faceworkers may act to defend themselves against the increasing area and complexity of their work, the dangers and demands of engaging in multiprofessional teamworking, uncertainties associated with including users and carers in decision-making and the interference of institutional managers whose knowledge and understanding of complex roles and functions may be limited (Laungani and Williams, 1997). From what has already been discussed in the previous chapters of this book the most valued aspect of the user/carer interface is that of the helping relationship, the compact between individual faceworkers and their clients. This, it seems, is the most valued aspect of collaboration and the one that needs most protection from the controlling influences of both the group or team and any dysfunctional institutional behaviours.

Before moving to explore these deeper issues it is interesting to note a further aspect of the carers' story about the Nutrition Project.

The Nutrition Project

Carer:
What happened was that the staff and the managers decided to work together on a project to see if the nutritional needs of patients could be met much better. What they did was arranged for staff to lay in bed and have someone feed them. They also got staff to pretend that they could not swallow. Then they brought in the speech therapist who also looks after swallowing and the physiotherapists to help people who could not use their hands properly. Then they tied up the hands of some people and got them to talk about what it was like to only have one hand to feed yourself. What was good about this was that we were invited to do the same things and to join in with the training. We were

in partnership with the staff and we felt that we had been able to make a contribution. This is still going on, we go in sometimes and help with more new staff and new patients to help with their nutrition.

This part of the story reflects the issues identified by Sally Hornby when she points to the effects of open communication and participative discussions during which good 'fellow-feelings' can be developed, as in the example of Mrs Smith, the social worker and the therapist (pages 165–166). It appears that there was little projection outside of the group, but rather a facing up to negative feelings, an overcoming of reluctance to share the domain of expertise with carers and a strengthening of fellow-feeling across the group. The identity boundaries of staff (faceworkers), managers, carers and users were maintained, otherwise they could not have contributed from their perspectives and their expertise. However, a wider sense of belonging to a bounded project has emerged; the expression of pleasure at being included and having a contribution to make is evident from the enthusiasm of the story-teller, who is herself a carer.

Drivers for change: threats to individuals and groups

Various drivers for the development of a local, multiprofessional partnership that included the carers can be detected from the carer's story. The first driver was that the faceworkers were presented with evidence of failure and with the possibility of a formal, damaging complaint from a carer in the interests of the user. The implications of such an incident were considerable. While the more obvious legal and professional aspects of the situation posed the risk of disciplinary action that could have resulted in individuals losing their jobs or membership of working teams, other aspects of the situation also posed considerable threats. These included perceived threats to the self-esteem and self-concept of individuals, to those of the group and to experiences of being in valued helping relationships with users and their carers, which could now be seen by others as ineffectual and weak. The shock of realising that the team had lost sight of their main purpose, to serve the needs of the clients, together with the sense of having failed to meet a most obvious and basic need of their clients, must have been considerable. However, rather than projecting any negative feelings towards the managers or other representatives of the organisation they began to look positively at themselves. The local multiprofessional team invested time, energy and financial resources into an open learning exercise involving trans-boundary communication, the sharing of perspectives and the development of ideas. The process would have included respect for each others' expertise, a telling realisation that the needs of the clients had been inexplicably missed in the rushed and wearing delivery of fast but ineffective services, and a move towards including carers and users in a learning team.

Drivers for change: motivational rewards

Other drivers from the case study include motivating rewards: the retention of self-esteem and self-concept, both of the individuals and the group of faceworkers, was crucial. Without this the team could have disintegrated, and helping relationships been further damaged as a consequence. Retaining team-based helping relationships, which had been established through the psycho-social interactions of individuals, was essential. In order to achieve this the members had to consider new perspectives and new ways of changing their interactive behaviours towards each other and to their clients. The amount of time, energy and other resources needed to achieve this can only be imagined but what is clear is that the outcomes, in terms of the enriching of both team interactions and the care of clients, were much improved.

The use of rewarding and informative learning strategies at ground level in improving individual and team performances could have an impact on organisational performance across many humane institutions in health and social care (Senge, 1990; Dechant et al, 1993). The example of the nutrition project is one among many that provides a model of transboundary, inclusive, collaborative care and suggests that there is considerable potential for higher levels of integration of practice, more satisfying roles for faceworkers and the maintenance of effective helping relationships. Sharing examples of such good practice could enable others to be aware of deficiencies in services long before situations deteriorate sufficiently to provide grounds for complaints. However, more attention needs to be paid to the underlying assumption that managerial or organisational practices contribute to faceworkers not being able to provide optimal care at all times.

Defining the task

Menzies Lyth (1988) pointed out that professional workers are often ambitious in what they would like to do for their clients, and therefore tend to define the tasks of institutions on fairly ambitious terms. Unlike profit-making institutions, which go bankrupt and fail if they set objectives beyond their means, humane institutions can often survive in this state even if they are not functioning well. In separate institutions staff tend to pursue adequate interventions for total populations as an end in itself without relating the defined task or objective to possible means; or they may not be in a position to do so. The result is chronic overwork, chronic disappointment in results, low satisfaction, high stress, and fruitless struggles with resource-dispensing authorities.

Humane institutions have difficulties in defining their tasks. For example, defining the purpose or primary task of prisons can be difficult. Primary tasks, in that example, may be interpreted variously as punitive, custodial or therapeutic. Another example is the primary task of schools: the definition of 'education' is variously interpreted as the transmission of information; preparation for future employment; or the socialisation of the nation's young. In other words humane institutions have multiple objectives and can sometimes be seen as examples of confusion and flux.

The multiplicity of interpretations of the primary tasks for humane institutions can lead to inadvertent anti-task or negative organisational learning if the organisation fails to be realistically orientated to the complexities of the needs of users, faceworkers and the carers because of societal and political pressures to perform against specific sets of criteria. One example could be the well-defined aims and objectives of integrated planning for quality in the NHS as presented in papers such as 'The New NHS: Modern and Dependable' (Secretary of State, 1997). The ideal of the 'third way' of running the NHS as a system 'based on partnership and driven by performance' — is a move away from outright competition towards a more collaborative approach (NHS Modern, Dependable, 1997 pages 10 and 11) . We have already seen that collaboration is not an easy concept to achieve. Although one of the six key principles from the document points to a level of local responsibility with doctors and nurses in the driving seat it is unlikely to succeed unless there is an open, participative management style at ground level practice. This suggests that information, based on comprehensive assessments of material, financial and human resource factors, is required for feeding into a consultative and negotiated process of faceworker–managerial dialogue. There are no directions for guiding this very human endeavour and so the aims may be seen as self-defeating; an extra load of rhetoric and vague ideas being imposed on an already over-stretched staffing structure.

Likewise the aims of 'clinical governance' outlined in 'The new NHS: Modern – Dependable' (1997) and in the consultation paper 'Clinical Governance – Quality in the new NHS' (NHS Executive 1999) of 'making sure that healthcare organisations develop cultures, systems and ways of working which assure that the quality of care is at the heart of the business of all organisations – at every level' could be seen as a set of overarching concepts and impositions, lacking details of how the aims are to be achieved, and with little attention being paid to the dynamics of the social structures required to implement them.

In either case little recognition is offered to the ground level faceworker and their need to maintain helping relationships. In both examples much emphasis is placed on board-room decision-making and the role of NHS trusts/consortia and local authorities. While these are very necessary organisational structures and roles through which to address the key principles of change, the location of decision-making in board rooms and governing bodies' offices creates limitations on collaborative dialogue between managers and ground level faceworkers. Local involvement is encouraged throughout these policy documents but there is sparse evidence of upward communication from the user/faceworker interface. The complexity of the task, as viewed from the interface with clients, needs to be defined at that lowest level rather than by broad aims that are often unrealistic and unrelated to resource objectives at board level. Indeed, the local initiatives taken by the staff in the example above achieved more in practice than 'top-down' impositions of ambitious objective-setting that are ultimately beyond the means of achievement by the ground-level staff.

So long as board-room level of decision-making, however 'local', remains widely divergent from the complexity of ground level work policies and guidance it will be seen as half-hearted, and its achievements as negligible (Hudson, 2000). Dialogue between faceworkers and decision-makers at board-room level is essential if the complex and rapidly changing interface of user and carer service is to be understood and managed at the ground level. Failure on the part of managers and faceworkers to enter into dialogue can lead to managers planning superficial solutions to much deeper problems.

Dysfunctional organisational learning

The potential failure of managers to recognise the realities and complexities of situations faced by faceworkers can cause increasing pressure on faceworkers themselves. For example, if managers are unaware of the efforts required of faceworkers to build relationships with more than one client (for example, children-parents or patients-carers), cope with uncertainties, dilemmas, increasing levels of responsibility and in the changing nature of the boundaries of professional control, they will not be in a position to collaborate at the managerial/faceworker interface or be able to encourage others to achieve the primary, humane task of the organisation. Pressures on managers to turn their attention towards externally generated criteria for performance, and to meeting political/legal goals, can lead to defensive behaviours and dysfunctional organisational learning because such redirection prevents them from meeting their own primary goals.

The following case study illustrates some of these points.

Betty, confusion, dependency and control

Betty is an elderly, frail and slightly confused lady, with a tendency to leave her money lying around in full view of everyone. She is in very obvious danger of losing it or having it stolen. A concerned neighbour contacted Social Services without Betty's permission and Social Services acted on the information to set up a new system of organising Betty's benefit payments. Social Services now manage the payment of bills and control the flow of cash by taking her pension book and rearranging other cash payments. Betty is exceedingly angry at having her pension book taken away, at the loss of her independence and at the sense of being diminished as a human being. Consequently, Betty refuses any other kinds of help from Social Services. She feels that they will take control over everything and she refuses to see the need for further assistance or accept any further help because 'blinded' by her anger.

Betty's case illustrates the point that the primary task for some institutions increasingly appears to be the defence of their own departments and their own resources. These institutions will hide behind the limitations of their separate budgets and even appeal to the law when under attack. These defensive attitudes have enormous implications for face-to-face relation-ships and can lead to expressions of angry behaviours on several fronts. The interests of the institutions appeared to be focused on conserving their own funds and saving 'their' money from being wasted. In the above situation concerns on the part of social services led to defensive behaviour involving the professionals taking control which, in turn, led to anger on the part of the client and her rejection of any further attempts to help her. The purpose of social services in terms of their wider primary task was therefore defeated.

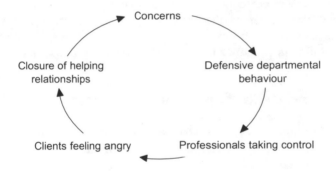

Fig. 16.1 The cycle of dysfunctional learning

In terms of efficient use of resources failure to achieve the primary task of enabling Betty to be effectively independent meant that new interventions had to be devised and implemented. New practices take more time and place even greater demands on the use of resources, so they need to be questioned carefully. If practices are not sufficiently questioned the organi-sation learns in a negative fashion as these practices become habitual and are internalised as the normal response of the system. In these cases a spiral of defensive decisions and practices leads to ever more negative effects in terms of the primary task and the thwarting of the original purposes of the helping system. The example of Betty illustrates how such a spiral can develop as the reduction of her independence led to increasing levels of hostility and increasing levels of rejection on her part of further helping interventions.

Drivers to defend organisations can be explained in terms of group dynamics, group behaviours and organisational theories. Significant elements of the collective subconscious thoughts and feelings of individuals, expressed in everyday interactive language and behaviours, can manifest themselves in the institutional norms that emerge within groups over time and which act to regulate the system (Vickers, 1981). Such 'norming' behaviours can reveal themselves in the expectations of organisations and can be expressed as the criteria for success or failure by the consensus of the whole institution as it attempts to define its purpose or domain.

The psychosocial processes of norming contrast with the rationality required to map the demands placed on health and social care services. In functioning within unpredictable environments humane institutions face many uncertainties, such as the number of people who will experience heart disease or cancer in a given time period, or how many families will need specialist help from social services. These uncertainties can create profound anxieties about predicting the success or failure of the institution. The criteria for success or failure, however, may not be unitary, given, or attainable in objective terms; it may only be realised by the organisation succeeding in what it was designed to do. Superficial problem definitions, for humane institutions, may therefore hide much more profound issues associated with the values, beliefs and norms of those who constitute the user/faceworker interface and their anxieties to succeed at this level of operations.

Surface and deep, significant problems

Bain (1982) gives an example of superficial problem definition and deeper, more significant organisational issues. In his work with a computer processing company he observed what was being said in a group he was interviewing and what appeared when the situation was explored in a much deeper fashion. He heard a great deal about what the operators felt was wrong with their life at work and what action was required to put it right; for example, more flexible hours, being allowed to chat as they might in an office job, free tea and coffee, and so on. Bain felt that these expressions were superficial and that there was something much more significant concerning the job itself and the workers' job-centred experiences. With Bain's help the workers discussed their jobs and experiences. A rather terrible picture emerged from their disclosures: loss of a sense of self or fears of such a loss; loss of awareness of what was going on although they continued to function; feelings of being automata, or like the machines they worked with, and irritation, alienation, boredom, and depersonalisation. This account was much more convincing and suggested that the action needed to ameliorate matters should be directed at the work situation itself and not at the fringe benefits.

Managers and planners run the risk of failing to engage in meaningful dialogue with faceworkers and hence failing to arrive at real diagnoses of problems. Remedies to address fringe benefits or superficial expressions of disquiet are often instituted repetitively and found to be ineffectual time and time again while the core problem remains virtually untouched. Examples of this include making pay awards to nurses, committed and highly motivated workers. While they welcome this kind of reward, nurses also need to feel that the complex nature of their work is fully appreciated and that strategic planning takes account of this in the context of the huge numbers of variables nurses (and other faceworkers) need to address in meeting users' needs.

The following case illustrates this point from the perspective of social services.

Open social services department offices

Strategic planning in one Local Authority Social Service Department identified three, out of numerous, local offices as being the only ones 'open' to the general public. The other offices, across the county, would continue to run but with no duty social work cover. Clients however, still found their way to these offices, often in very distressed states only to find administrative office staff who were unable to help them. The clients' frustrations were often expressed towards the staff in the office who could only offer to transmit requests by telephone to another office.

The clients' distress left the administrative staff in the 'non-open' offices feeling demotivated, demoralised and deskilled since they were left in a position of not being able to address the immediate and distressing situations brought to them. Special training sessions for the staff were set up in order to enable them to deal with clients' problems in a competent and professional manner. Some attention was paid to how they felt about the situation but the underlying issue of there being no qualified and experienced social workers available was not addressed so the staff continued to feel alienated from the organisation and inadequate in dealing with clients' problems.

Chapter 17 provides an example of a long-term collaborative partnership with a user and his family, the nature of the changing culture that accompanied the relationship and lessons for future practice. A second case study illustrates how the valued faceworker-user interface is protected by both individuals and groups by evasion of the guidelines and legal precedents set by authorities who remain distant from ground level practices.

Chapter 17
The Environment of Collaborative Care

Introduction

In this chapter the authors discuss potential hindrances to collaborative practice at the ground level, unintentionally derived from higher levels of organisational and institutional structures. Themes arising from the demands for quality assurance, clinical audit and clinical governance have been discussed in Chapter 16. The regulatory mechanisms implied by these concepts are rational and necessary, but the language and focus appear to be concentrated more on the needs of bureaucratic institutions than on the needs of faceworkers dealing with the day-to-day complexities at the user and carer interface.

Impressive examples of successful collaborations, in which such hindrances have been overcome by groups and individuals interacting across the boundaries of profession or speciality, are drawn from further case studies. Although the details of how these processes came to be so successful are not given they all have the same drivers for change, concern to develop better helping relationships with users and carers; and satisfying roles for the ground-level faceworkers themselves. To these could be added the satisfaction of collaborating successfully with the managers and decision-makers within organisations.

Achieving collaborative integration of care

Individual faceworkers can feel constrained in their ability to meet the needs of users and carers by the broad policies, aims and objectives of their local organisation or agencies, especially when it comes to the distribution of resources. While the faceworker may be able, either alone or as a team, to assess users' and carers' needs and continue to develop the necessary critical thinking and expertise to meet them, they may still fail at the first hurdle of limitations in staffing, lack of time and lack of material resources to meet those needs according to their personal, professional and group standards. One cause of this operational difficulty has already been identified as the failure to link organisational objectives to the resources necessary to achieve them. This failure can be worsened if objective performance criteria, which have been established through processes such as clinical audit, are in place. Unless such audits are managed well they can contribute to a climate of tension and fear of failure in the faceworker.

The security and identities of faceworkers are woven into the familiar and stable order of things within the context of their local and professional organisations. The social organisation in which faceworkers find themselves, including aspects of accepted, embedded power, are made explicit in the natural running of day-to-day systems and processes. Familiar socialisation patterns, illustrated in the use of power in decision-making, policy formation and emergent hierarchies within groups, can be challenged if the expert power of faceworkers' day-to-day monitoring of changing and complex situations is not incorporated into new and adaptable patterns of work.

> "It can be difficult to challenge the way things are or even to recognise in the first place that what one is presented with is an established pattern of power relations and not some immutable facet of social reality. It is clearly in the best interests of those who possess power if the unequal distribution of power is accepted, taken for granted, not challenged, accepted, invisible."
>
> (Buchanan and Badman, 1999, p. 55)

The faceworker brings their accepted understanding of the organisational contexts in which they work to their first encounter with the users and clients. As soon as they begin to develop a relationship of helping and the process of assessing the users' and carers' troubles they can become aware of the constraints that some organisational contexts exert. The task of feeding information about users' and carers' requirements back into power structures and patterns of work can be difficult, especially when the faceworker needs to challenge the resource power of the decision-makers higher up in the organisation. Faceworkers can feel powerless in the face of existing organisational structures, systems and procedures, especially if what they have discovered at the assessment stages with users and carers suggests a need for organisational change.

Complexities of assessment

In Chapter 5 Sally Hornby reflects on the nature of assessment and the various perspectives that contribute to an alignment of the subjective views of the user and the more objective views of the faceworker (page 53). Assessment, she points out, has two fundamental objectives: to decide on the most appropriate form of help; and to determine whether the face-worker or the agency can provide it. One of the complexities at the user–faceworker interface is identified here in that from the outset the faceworker needs to decide how far to go on their own authority and expertise and when to seek the help of other team members or experts. S/he has to decide the extent to which the subjective views of the user should be considered, and whether the assessment indicates that the situation is complicated by underlying psychological, personal or social troubles. S/he needs to decide if one or more agency, such as both health and social services, should be involved, and s/he may have to make these judgements on the basis of limited time and incomplete assessments. Moreover, as Sally Hornby points out, at times the responsibility which a faceworker has is not matched by adequate power to discharge it. The worker may lack either the necessary skills, material resources or authority to deal with a situation. Responsibility for this lack may be the faceworker's or it may belong higher up the line in professional training, management, policy-making or legislation (page 50).

While Sally Hornby's recommendation to consider MEA (*minimum essential assessment*) (page 53) is helpful, in that time constraints and users wishes always need to be considered, meeting the requirements of policies, guidelines and standards may present particular difficulties for faceworkers. The pressure to integrate one's personal values and judgements with those of the team and with those of external, organisational influences can create a sense of being overwhelmed with complexity and, in due course, with a sense of failure and fear.

Wider organisational influences

As well as problems in making assessments there is an increasing demand for the prediction and monitoring of outcomes in order to establish the relative effectiveness and efficiency of interventions (Muir-Grey, 1998) and present evidence of having met standards through the use of clinical audit (Baker et al 1999). Both the need to ensure that practice is based on the latest evidence, and that it meets the requirements of quality assurance initiatives and improvement programmes, can be challenging and stressful for faceworkers in the health and social care sectors today even though these demands are perfectly reasonable and rational. This is because they are underpinned by powerful psychosocial components such as the need for social and psychological safety in the group or team and in the organisation.

> *"Safety is the affective context within which people are more likely to engage in effective team working based on trust, acceptance, humour, warmth and support. Together these lead to the involvement, commitment and creativity of team members in team functioning in a positive climate"*

> *McCrea in Baker et al (1999) p. 124*

In terms of the helping relationship at the faceworker/user interface, and in particular the complexities of assessment of users' troubles, the need for psychosocial safety including respect for the faceworker's judgements and decisions by his or her colleagues, is paramount. Nowadays faceworkers consulting with others may not only be exposed to criticism of incompetence, as in the case of Mrs Smith (page 165), but also to the conflicting demands of formal clinical audit programmes.

McCrea (1999) suggests that one obstacle to health care quality management is that, compared with most manufacturing or service operations, health care outcomes are difficult to define, measure and control. McCrea points out that it is a popular but peculiar belief that health and social care practitioners control outcomes and that in these kinds of care there are no accidents and no complexities (especially those coming from user, carer and volunteer contributions to integrated care), only physicians and nurses who make mistakes and are therefore incompetent. Such a view can lead to a climate of fear and blame in which staff are afraid that their peers will think less of them when outcomes are disappointing. McCrea quotes Deming (1986) in saying that patient outcomes, good or bad, are typically seen as being due to provider skill alone. By contrast, in industry at least 80% of defects are due to management and the system it has created, while fewer than 20% are directly attributable to worker mistakes. There is little recognition of the difference between system failures and those directly attributable to the faceworker in health and social care. The management process is rarely blamed and even when it is investigated it is generally the practitioner who is put on the line.

The obstacle of fear

The obstacle of fear arises from the psychological defences that physicians, nurses, social workers and other members of the multidisciplinary team construct. There are many reasons why such individual defences arise including fear of rejection, fear of powerlessness, fear of social neglect, fear of isolation and fear of failing to deliver adequate services because of time constraints. In instances of team-working these negative forces may be balanced by positive forces such as camaraderie, empowerment and recognition. One way to reinforce the positive and reduce the negative factors includes the use of steps that pose no direct threats to individuals, such as regular meetings to define those processes and outcomes that constitute high quality care, and raise awareness of wider quality issues.

Overcoming defensive behaviours

There are many instances of teams of health care practitioners learning to work together in non-threatening forums. Likewise teams of social care practitioners have learned to do the same. They each work to share their common objectives and to decide on the most efficient use of limited resources. Often they will define their domains of care very carefully with an eye to ensuring that their specific domains are not encroached on, and even offload some aspects of care on to alternative teams or authorities. The following example illustrates how attempts to offload responsibility on to another authority led to three different outcomes, a legal case-law precedent, ground-level collaborative practice that went beyond the current requirements of the law, and an effect on users who did not necessarily benefit from the enhanced collaboration.

Health Authorities and Social Services: who should pay for nursing homes in the community?

In one county social services and the health authority have been increasingly working together to provide services to people with disabilities living in the community. At the same time the health authority had developed stringent criteria for judging when a patient would get needed nursing home care, which was fully funded by the NHS. As a result social services, using means testing, were funding all but a handful. This was very expensive for social services and meant that some very disabled people had to pay for their own care.

In July 1999 the Court of Appeal decided that social services responsibility for nursing care was limited and that health authorities would have to fully fund a substantial proportion of the people who had previously paid for their care or who had been means tested.

The judgement could have led to a rapid move by social services to remove the funding which the decision had indicated they should not have been making. Instead the management kept the matter low key. They did not seek to have the health authority redraft the suspect criteria. They had been working closely with the health authority and saw that if health had to take over payment for a large number of nursing home placements they would have to stop paying for other essential services, which would have caused disruption.

This spirit of partnership had an obvious valuable effect. The other side of it though was that a large number of people continued to be charged substantial sums, which they should not have paid. The close relationship that developed between health and social services prevented disruption, but at a cost to some service users.

Reformulating the boundaries

Several factors in this scenario are worth mentioning. The first is that by some mysterious process the boundaries of both teams had become more permeable and exchanges of perspectives, values, expertise and objectives apparently flowed in both directions across the boundaries. Secondly, the overall purpose of the authority on one side or the other was managed, presumably through enhanced consultation or negotiation. However, apparently neither the health authority nor social services succeeded in avoiding the team-absorption that tends to create dangers for team-working as discussed in Chapter 16. They still failed to meet the needs of some people with disabilities despite their collaborative action. In terms of the rewarding achievements of establishing satisfying relationships, and of meeting a wider set of organisational purposes than the limited perspective of costs, they succeeded; but in terms of the wider goals of user-carer focused care it appears they were not so successful.

Moving towards collaborative integration of services

Another example of collaborative, integrated services arose from discussions in a focus group with a carers' forum. This is a story covering 30 years and involving social services, the health authority, services for mental health and a family of carers with a son who has learning disabilities. The following extract is taken from part of the transcript of the discussion with the carer Paula Grey.

Paula: experiences of power domination, poor communication and improvements in teamworking over time

I think it is partnership that matters and getting people together to discuss all the issues because so often work gets duplicated which is a waste of time and effort. My son, who attended a day centre, began to have behavioural problems. A psychiatrist and a psychologist spent time with him but it was only after Jim (my son) was given a care manager that things began to happen. She pulled things together and arranged meetings of everyone concerned with Jim's care including his key worker at the day centre, his GP and ourselves. The care manager also spent time with Jim at the day centre where she felt he would be most comfortable with meeting her. That was what was needed – one person who can pull things together – who is taking a lead. The funding issues – that was of course very difficult – virtually impossible to get health people together but when you try to pull in social services it is difficult. Luckily, with learning disabilities the health side was 'on tap'. The psychologist, psychiatrist and doctor were all involved much more.

The above extract captures key aspects of end-point learning that had taken place over many years. The carer's experiences at the inception of care, some 30 years beforehand, had been very different. She had felt disempowered and marginalised. She felt that her views were unimportant, she was not part of the decision-making process and that the professionals were taking control. She had experienced anything but 'partnership' in her contacts with both health and social services. Above all, she felt that her deep knowledge of her own, her husband's and her son's needs were being ignored. She was very fearful that without this 'inside' knowledge the plans for her son's care could go horribly wrong for years to come. The actions she took and the outcomes, in terms of enhanced teamwork and partnership with the family, are captured in the following extract of an interview with her about the situation.

INTERVIEWER: "If you think back now are there things that you wish you had known earlier or could you suggest how the authorities could have handled things differently?"

PAULA: "Get and give a real diagnosis of what is going on. They should get a real diagnosis of what the problems are and tell the parents – tell the parents exactly what the problem is but don't go too far into the future and say that this means that in nineteen years or so this or that will be the problem.

INTERVIEWER: "You mentioned a couple of very unpleasant things people told you then. Could you say again what these were?"

PAULA: "At the school (for learning disabilities) the head teacher told us 'He'll never be independent' which, I mean, times have changed but they meant that it would go on into the future.

INTERVIEWER: "And they said that to you – straight out?"

PAULA: "Yes, it was just said like that. There was a psychiatrist who since has been employed by the education service – and his wife was a teacher at the school. Jim had pulled someone or done something while they were playing and they said that he was a danger to other people and should be in an institution. We were both shocked by this statement. I was in tears – tears of anger. Making such a decision after spending little time with Jim and with little evidence to support it seemed to me to be unforgivable.

INTERVIEWER: "What caused you to be so angry?"

PAULA: "It could have affected all his life. We heard that this man was leaving the school psychiatry service for one with adults. At least he would not be able to dismiss children and their futures.

INTERVIEWER: "There appear to be two kinds of people making judgements on very slim evidence?

PAULA: "There was a suggestion at one time that the Rudolf Steiner schools would be a possibility but I said 'No'. I just dug my heels in because I just didn't think it was right that all people with learning disabilities should be just lumped together even in a beautiful country setting miles from anywhere and so I said 'No'. Jim and my husband went to look at it but I refused to go – I said they could look at it but I was not going to even consider letting him go there. In retrospect I think I was right to do this as things have turned out because had he gone there he would have been in a community of learning disabilities people and then he would have been institutionalised no matter what the community was like. I am convinced I was right with that but I was made to feel I was not right but I dug my heels in."

INTERVIEWER: "Are there some morals you would like to draw from these experiences – that could perhaps be shared with others?"

PAULA: "Yes, I think there has to be much more co-operation and anything that is said to parents has to be considered (carefully). They must not make predictions about what is going to happen in five or ten years time. Because so many things change everyone has to have an open mind. Like that psychiatrist, he wasn't approaching it with an open mind – he'd heard a tale from someone. They have to go into it as though they know nothing. It is OK to read notes but that is just to keep some things in mind and maybe to refer to someone else who is in a position to know the situation. They should realise that they can make a great difference to someone's life and shouldn't make decisions quickly. What they pass on to parents has to be very considered and positive – as positive as can be – and honest because parents have got to come to terms with these things sometimes and it doesn't help if someone lies and says 'Oh it'll be all right in a year' – that doesn't help."

INTERVIEWER: "You are saying that honesty comes first, that honesty has to be reflected in a measured way?"

PAULA: "Yes, there are all sorts of ways of telling people bad news – you can tell them in a sympathetic way – an understanding way – and I think this isn't often done."

INTERVIEWER: "You can identify a positive aspect of this?"

PAULA: "Oh yes, we are getting to that now. People with Down's Syndrome were not being treated as well as they might be in the 1950s and 1960s. Someone was told by a consultant at that time that of course, they – meaning the hospital – would prefer to spend £10,000 on a normal person and this sort of thing. It is unforgivable, you know, you can't tell parents that – well you can, but you shouldn't.

In the 1970s a friend of mine took her son who had Down's Syndrome to the doctor and he said, 'I don't know why you're complaining, they are usually dead by the time they are 20 anyway' and she was devastated. She knew something was wrong, her son's hair was very poor and falling out, his skin went scaly and he was losing weight. My husband knew another doctor and my friend took her son there – he actually diagnosed it and got him into hospital – they later found out from research that he had a gluten thing that affected him very badly but no-one had pinned this down. He started to grow into a young man and he is in his 50s now."

INTERVIEWER: "Your story points to morals from several points of view. Are you saying that the quality of work isn't just as we sometimes think – that we need more resources or different skills – what do you think?"

PAULA: "I think what is so important is that people going into this sort of thing (learning disabilities) should know that quality is very important – the thoughtfulness of trying to put yourself in the place of the person who is hearing bad news and not making snap judgements. You can't do this about people."

INTERVIEWER: "Things did begin to turn around and get much better later?"

PAULA: "There was no contact with psychiatric services during the 1980s. The family GPs were understanding and as Jim began to show signs of epilepsy he had tests arranged by the school doctor who was very helpful and considerate. She asked for the test to be carried out in as informal way as possible – no white coats in sight. In 1994 Jim began to show signs that all was not well. Once again the psychologist and psychiatrist were involved but this time we were also involved and given suggestions of ways in which we could help. Some other consultants seemed unable to understand how to treat people with learning disabilities but there were exceptions. Once a care manager had been allocated and after she had spent time with Jim there were decisions made about his care with input from the psychologist and ourselves. The care manager had access to funding and after viewing several options it was decided that the right place was group home with staff who understood Jim's problems and were trained to help him. There he was encouraged to say what he wanted in his life and we were asked our views on his care. We were kept informed of progress and visited regularly. Jim came to stay with us for weekends and Christmas. After a time in the group home Jim called a meeting of people who could help him achieve his dream of his own home. We all listened to him and decided there was a way to do this. Just over a year and many meetings later Jim moved into a house he had chosen to buy in partnership with a housing association. He has twenty-four-hour support funded by social services. His GP and psychiatrist work with his care managers on health matters such as medications. We live just five minutes away and are members of his support circle. Jim makes all the house rules and decisions on the way he lives and what he does. He is in control of his own life. Without collaboration by many people from different agencies this could not have happened."

The extract illustrates how the organisational cultures and power distributions within them have changed, in this instance, over time. The synthesis of users' and carers' voices with those of the immediate faceworkers and those in the wider organisational context have led eventually, after several decades, to a collaborative integrated care approach that appears to meet the objectives of all parties through an accommodation of views. How this came about remains a mysterious process but Paula did provide some further insights into cause-and-effect relationships. The most effective agent in precipitating the change was the care manager. When this person took a lead role and actively brought the various parties together 'things started to go then'. Apparently things did not continue to 'go' with a change of manager, but when the same ideas were reinstated with another visionary manager it was with the same positive effect. This implies that the selection of competent and confident leaders in key positions such as care managers will make a considerable difference in the achievement of collaborative, integrated care in the future. One aspect of developing such leaders lies in the potential of new training programmes such as joint degrees in learning disability nursing and social work. Such programmes could lead to enhanced trans-boundary collaboration and enhanced dialogue between professional groups, managerial strategic planners and ground-level practice.

The impact of organisational structures and dynamics on collaborative care

Strauss *et al.* (1973) comment that organisations are not always the happy, harmonious, collaborative communities that many management texts imply, but are more appropriately viewed from a 'negotiated order' perspective. When decision trails are tracked it can be seen that they are typically the results of bargaining, trading and compromising between many participants, each engaged in obtaining the best deal for their interests. Paula presents her case for a wider distribution of information and the power to contribute to decision-making on behalf of her son, indeed she advocates and welcomes the inclusion of her son's own opinions into decisions regarding his care. The specialists she encountered earlier in her story used their expert power to control the decision-making processes regarding the future life-style of her son, indeed the quality of his life for years to come. The split between agencies appeared at one time to contribute to powerlessness among those who had the best chances of providing appropriate care but the most powerful person, in terms of moving things forward, was the care manager. This was someone who entered centre stage at a later date and represents one aspect of a movement towards client-centred collaborative care.

It appears that some organisations can constrain their members and restrict creative developments from taking place. However, Tushman (1977) suggests that the organisational structures we see around us develop from political tensions between individual members and groups or coalitions. Political processes arise not because of individual or group perversity, but because of the nature of organisational interactions and decision-making under uncertainty. Bureaucratic methods and bureaucratic organisations are the least well equipped to deal with uncertainties and hence would be those most likely to impose constraining influences on workers at ground-level practice.

"If decisions must be made without sufficient information or in the face of diverse goals, then non-bureaucratic methods must evolve to attend to the

*differences in preferences, values, and beliefs about cause and effect
relations. If even the most objective issues are open to multiple interpretations, and if organisational participants often derive different
meanings from the same information base, then bureaucratic decision-
making procedures will unambiguously decide only a limited set of organisational decisions."*

(Tushman, 1977, p.212)

Schein (1988) suggested that the problems inherent in working in an
organisation are further complicated by the changing environment of the
organisation itself. The tremendous growth of technology and the changing
norms about priorities, such as enhanced quality improvement programmes, evidence-based care and ensuring effective treatments for more
people in ever-tightening time frames, all contribute to 'turbulence' in the
working environment of the faceworker. These changes require a different
kind of capacity to respond on the part of organisations as well as individual
faceworkers. Systems models offer some ideas on how complex, open
organisations work. For example, the idea of socio-technical systems,
defined by studies conducted at the Tavistock Institute in London, suggest
that relationships between tasks and those who perform them must be
considered in the work of productive organisations. In the case of faceworkers such relationships could be illustrated in notions of critical practice,
where the faceworker might seek out information from systematic reviews
and other sources of evidence from a research-based environment and
import new ideas into his/her individual practice. Faceworkers, would,
however, hold expectations that they would be supported by their organisational structures and managers in the implementation of changes in
practice.

*'Not only must the organisation deal with the demands and constraints
imposed by the environment in terms of raw materials, money and consumer preferences, it must also deal with the expectations, values and
norms of its members. Employees' capacities, preferences and expectations of employers are, from this point of view, not merely "givens," but
factors that are undoubtedly influenced by the nature of the job and the
organisational structure they come up against. Consequently, one cannot
solve work problems merely by better selection or training techniques.
Rather, the initial design of the organisation must take into account both
the nature of the job (the technical system) and the nature of the people
(who perform it) – (the social system)'*

(Schein, 1998, p. 193).

The current environment of health and welfare services is increasingly affected by internal and external turbulence. The uncertainties that these create will have an impact on the faceworker and the helping relationship at the ground level of practice. They may adversely affect faceworkers' sense of identity and role security and so create a greater need for measures to deal with high levels of stress. Bureaucratic rules and regulations will fail to meet these needs; participative, open management styles might succeed. The perceptions, values and expertise of ground-level faceworkers, including users and carers as central to the helping compact norms, may then be incorporated into decision-making and planning at all levels of the organisation. Utopian and idealistic as this may sound, the experiences of Betty and Paula suggest that this collaborative method is a more successful way to go. Paula's example shows that it is possible, and it is essential if issues of quality assurance, clinical governance and consumer satisfaction are to be met.

Chapter 18
The Three Collaborative Frameworks

Introduction

In this chapter the authors revisit the framework adopted by Sally Hornby in the earlier chapters of this book. In the first part the concepts of the help-compact and helping relationships are revisited and applied to the interface between faceworkers and their managers or organisations. It is suggested that the helping role, as defined by Sally Hornby, can be extended in order to enable faceworkers to manage the complexities of the help-compact with users and carers. Recent announcements from government sources appear to suggest that the knowledge and expertise of faceworkers will be brought to bear in the form of advice at the executive level of NHS strategic planning. It is suggested that a negotiated ordering of services across the boundaries of agencies and authorities would enable the voices of users and carers to be heard at ground level, and incorporated into the advice being given to planners. These relational aspects of working are seen to enhance the idea of the help-compact at higher levels in the organisation of services.

In the second part the structures and resource pools described by Sally Hornby are revisited in relation to current changes in the organisation of services. Relational aspects of ground-level work are draining in terms of their emotional content for faceworkers handling features such as risk-taking and uncertainties for both themselves and their clients. This kind of work is stressful, but there are other kinds of stress arising from the changing environment of the organisation. Restructuring, changes in methods of working and changes in interprofessional relationships can cause staff to experience feelings akin to grief. It is suggested that the helping relationship, from a managerial perspective, could be used to develop ways of helping faceworkers to deal with such manifestations of stress. This would further enable them to continue to develop valued helping relationships with their clients.

In the third part the authors reconsider the domain and functioning of faceworkers in the light of the organisational context of collaboration, which is a central part of the focus of Part III. The domains of faceworkers in both health and social care are more mobile than in the past and often it is the faceworker him/herself who defines both the boundary and the location of their functioning. The chapter closes with a consideration of the impact these changes have on collaborative practice.

Revisiting collaborative framework I: provision of help and helping relationships

The distinction between the concepts of 'caring' and 'helping' at the face-worker–user interface can also be made at the faceworker–organisational level of relationship. In Chapter 4 Sally Hornby describes caring as looking after, with human concern, through tending and protecting. It implies a position of ability and responsibility in the carer, in relation to some lack of capacity in the user. Helping, in contrast, is described as assisting users to improve or at least maintain their situation, and does not imply an imbalance of capacity as does caring.

In terms of the faceworker–organisational level of relationship these terms can be reinterpreted as managerial helping for the operational level of the worker, or enabling the worker to perform the actual work of delivering care through the responsible use of managerial expertise and ability to control resources. Helping faceworkers to improve the situation for users and to maintain the helping relationship does not imply an imbalance of capacity, but a more egalitarian base of power distribution. This is based on respect for expertise, and recognition of the role of faceworkers in dealing with the complexities of ground-level work practices.

In 1999 there was a move, on the part of the government, to ensure that the knowledge and expertise of medical faceworkers influences the decision-making systems of civil servants and hence strategic planning processes. Alan Millburn, Secretary of State for Health, speaking on a BBC Radio Four programme (World at One, Wednesday 23 February 2000), explained a proposal to develop a board of doctors, nurses, primary care groups and health care managers to advise the central management board on future policies and strategies for health. The introduction of 'hands-on experience' at the executive level of decision-making is seen as essential for ensuring that some experience of the realities of ground-level practice is brought to bear on strategies.

There is now widespread agreement with the idea of frontline people needing a frontline role in the planning of services, even across party boundaries. The separation of hierarchical and managerial policy-making processes from the ways in which policies are implemented is seen as undesirable, even though some members of the board are fearful of the effects of blurring these boundaries. It appears that the time is ripe for a more negotiated ordering of services and for faceworker–planning dialogue.

A negotiated order of inputs into services

While the structure and location of caring agencies, from the voluntary sector to NHS trusts and consortia, varies from place to place they all have a system boundary across which negotiations with other agencies take place. This point has been made in previous chapters in the context of secondary and participatory collaboration (page 42). The suggestion made here is that the same notions apply across the boundaries of levels of hierarchies within an organisation such as between faceworkers and their managerial colleagues. Definitions of boundaries of organisations, groups and agencies are most often established through the shared ideologies, aims and objectives held by their members. Expectations, or norms, such as loyalties, standards and accountability, also contribute to the social identification of such groups and form the basis for sets of assumptions that can be made about behaviours.

Faceworkers and managers will make assumptions about each others' roles within agencies and organisations and these roles are mostly stable during times of continuity and unchanging conditions. However, during times of rapid change in response to both governmental policy and consumer expectations and demands, roles themselves change, and much more negotiation is required for effective and adaptive service provision. As with instances of inter-agency collaboration discussed in Chapter 4 so it is with the changing and complex connections between the boundaries of faceworkers and managers.

The role of helpers is also changing. Both informal carers, such as families and friends, and local carers, such as volunteers in informal community groups or charities, are now much more likely to wish to be considered as part of the formal caring system and be included within the boundary of the decision-making system. The personal relationship does not exclude family and friends from being part of the decision-making system; on the contrary their knowledge of the user's needs and preferences is of the greatest value in the planning and delivering of appropriate and effective care, as Paula's case illustrates (page 190).

Policy and practices encourage the presentation of troubles in locations that are more accessible and immediate than those of GPs' surgeries, accident and emergency departments or paramedical services. The new 'NHS Direct' services are an instance of these changes. The aim is to provide greater access to diagnosis and information on health matters. Although subsequent routing of users is still unclear, the intention is to relieve GP practices and accident and emergency departments of an ever-increasing load. The assumption is that more use will be made of the expertise of a range of alternative therapeutic agencies such as pharmacists, as well as local health services, but evidence of the effectiveness of these re-routings is still unknown.

Improved access to diagnosis may be helpful but in terms of establishing a help-compact, and achieving helping relationships, users and their troubles need to be seen in the context of their life situations and within a negotiated order of service provision. The help-compact requires input from the user, and involves consideration of their current relationships and a review of their current situation. Help offered outside of a help-compact raises questions about the effectiveness of easier access of the sort offered by 'NHS Direct' which can only focus on the immediate, (and usually physical) presenting conditions, and is unable to take into account underlying or concurrent troubles for the users.

Meaningful helping relationships

The relationship between the faceworker and user is multifaceted and the help-compact varies from case to case. For example, the help provided may be a single treatment or episode of enablement or it may involve several methods and instances integrated into a whole. The help-compact may still be one involving several faceworkers and agencies. This will require high levels of communication, negotiation and agreement across a number of inter-agency and organisational boundaries and between levels of hierarchy within agencies and groups.

Currently, the idea that the help-compact covers all kinds of methods of help and a range of resources is useful since it distinguishes between the help-compact and the helping task. The helping task refers solely to human resources; it is the sum of human activity and may include identification of the resources necessary for carrying out a particular help-compact. The discussion with Paula about the management of her son with learning disabilities in Chapter 17 provides an example. However, one of the main aspects of human resource inputs into the relationship is the part associated with sentiments and the emotional work that is part of the psychosocial domain.

As discussed on page 40, for every helping task there is a level of minimum essential collaboration or MEC. This means the minimum number of people with the necessary competence for the task using the minimum integration of material resources and the minimum amount of time to achieve it. This scientific and quantitative approach may be useful for the measurement of standards of care, quantities of time, material resources and the use of expensive experts, but as Sally Hornby pointed out in Chapter 4 the perfection of a help-compact is more akin to the art of cookery (page 40).

To 'confect' the whole, through the mixing of ingredient parts of the helping task, is an organic process whose success depends on the art of the creative 'cook'. It is not only the sum of the constituent parts which determines the quality of the help provided, but the way in which it has been confected – the proportions, the blending, the timing and the intensity of input over time. Confecting the ingredients of the helping relationship will include many aspects of psychosocial work with users and carers. In Chapter 6 Sally Hornby states that for faceworkers to internalise the feelings, relational patterns and attitudes of users is such a common phenomenon, that to find ways of either neutralising or making good use of this process is essential (page 65).

Confected work and managing anxiety and stress

In recent years the importance of attending to the emotional impact of what can be defined as 'confected work' has been emphasised, and is seen as essential by some authors if excessive levels of stress among workers is to be avoided (Laungani and Williams, 1997). Adopting patient- or client-focused care in a multiprofessional or multi-agency approach involves a holistic approach to caring that challenges current systems of practice, and, for some, their identity as professionals. Organisational change can in itself present deep problems of a philosophical nature for some faceworkers, and trigger many kinds of work-related stressors. Laungani and Williams cite one study of a joint health and social services project (James and Dewhurst 1995) that showed organisational change creating such a sense of loss and grief among staff that their reactions were as acute as if they had suffered a minor bereavement. For example, during conversations with social workers it transpired that the introduction of the care management role was seen by some of them as marking 'the death knell of social work as we know it'.

Marris (1998) points to a sense of ambivalence and loss at times of considerable change. Members of groups may mourn the loss of some familiar patterns of working or loss of identity, even if the sense of mourning is banished or denied for a time.

> *"The vitality of that response depends upon a commitment of purpose, which has already been given and cannot now be wished away, even though the relationships which incorporated it have been disrupted"*
>
> *(Marris, 1998, page 92)*

For the individual faceworker and for agencies and groups the continuity of relationships is highly valued, as well as the challenges of change. Threats to these relationships, whether at the level of user-carer interface with faceworkers, or at the interface between faceworkers and their managers or organisations, need constant attention if negative side-effects are not to occur. Recommendations include step-by-step analysis of the main stressors that impinge on job satisfaction, or tools such as the 'Job Stress Survey' (Speilberger and Reheiser, 1994, cited by Laungani and Williams 1997).

Revisiting collaborative framework II: structures and the resource pool

Avoidance of issues like those experienced in the psychosocial domain, such as loss, grief and ambivalence, is an insufficient response if collaborative care is to succeed. Faceworkers carry high levels of responsibility and are usually highly skilled and competent practitioners. Their self-image is usually high and they are aware of both the general nature of the role and the specificity of the personal components, such as commitment to the helping relationship. They are therefore vulnerable to demoralisation and demotivation if effective dialogue and communication patterns between them and those who control the resource pool necessary for them to carry out their work are missing.

Involvement with the users' situations can be draining for faceworkers for the reasons described above, and if support is only offered in terms of material resources it may not be sufficient to enable faceworkers to fulfil their role. Faceworkers need to adapt to the situations for users, and the structures and resource pools available for them must therefore be adaptive and responsive to their needs.

The following case study of a situation in 1999 involved a user, Mrs B, with a progressive degenerative disease. It illustrates something of the nature of emotional involvement and support required for collaborative multi-professional work.

The views are those of a care manager on the demands of collaboration in social work.

Mrs B, sufferer from a degenerative disease

> In discussing this case I would wish to demonstrate the complex issues around risk assessment and in allowing clients to determine the amount of statutory intervention without disempowerment. While working on this very difficult and complex case it was vital for me to work closely with other disciplines, in particular with the primary health care team and the care providers. At a later date I had to work closely with the juvenile justice team and police. Staying focused on and working with my client, respecting her decisions and supporting those decisions was sometimes very difficult. I had to deal with my own and others' value judgements.

The above extract confirms Sally Hornby's view that individual workers are in a strong position in determining role-relationships (page 99) and using their role to define helping methods. It is usually practitioners who hold the power-position in defining roles but users are seeking a more active part in this area, an attitude supported by this care manager. Greater user participation is demanded in the process of role definition and, if rightly used, clarifies the functions and responsibilities of the people concerned. The care manager also had to define her role in relation to other role-holders in the situation. She goes on to say:

> **W**e held a case conference organised by the Community Hospital. The primary nurse from the ward and the District Nurse were present along with the home care worker. The lady was looked after by her husband, Mr B, but there were anxieties about possible neglect, especially with food, and even abuse. The plan was for an occupational therapist to visit and discuss entry to the home via the doors. This would allow Mrs B to control who came in and out while Mr B was away. What was bothering me was that Mrs B seemed so powerless. I suppressed my scepticism about the situation on my first visit and handled the relationship building sensitively and well. In the first meeting I employed a task centred approach working in a well-defined role. I identified needs and worked towards a set of shared, agreed outcomes, i.e. frozen meals, microwave and so on.
>
> All the goals were met, the microwave arrived, the new doors were installed and the carer was coming in to help with the food. All the time I felt that I very much wanted to spend more time with Mrs B in order to get to know her and form some relationship with her. I was aware that she shared a lot of her fears and concerns with her carer – that she missed her husband who was "never around" and would often weep uncontrollable tears in her carer's arms. Also, it appeared that Mrs B's son was eating the meals, meeting with his friends in the house and possibly behaving illegally. The carers felt vulnerable in this situation and their concerns and feelings were taken very seriously. My action was to alert my line manager and arrange for a risk assessment as soon as possible. I discussed the issues with the home care manager and we set up a meeting with the home care unit manager, the home care co-ordinator and myself. Mrs B. was also subject to social isolation and was unable to maintain her own dependency in financial terms. There were serious breakdowns between the father and the son.
>
> We had to avoid hearsay and premature judgements and we needed to work closely with the primary health team, the care manager, the unit manager, the home care manager, the district nurse and the local GP. We were all concerned to conduct a careful risk assessment, a highly complex and difficult task for professionals and for multidisciplinary teams. Achieving personal choice, maximum independence, dignity and control may involve risk taking where there are possible undesirable outcomes as well as possible rewards.
>
> Needs assessment involved risk assessment but also included unmet needs. Advice and guidance for the user can so easily slip into coercion when workers are anxious about the effects of illness on users' abilities to make appropriate judgements about risks. An exchange model of assessment is not particularly helpful since it assumes that the worker has expertise in problem-solving and the user has expertise about the problem.

I had taken Mrs B to a Leonard Cheshire Home the previous week to see if she would like to go there for a period of respite care. We had a relationship of trust and I was able to ask her about her feelings. She said she was alright and had no problems. Mr B, she said, had improved recently and 'No, she did not want to have her benefits book'. Although it was appropriate to take her to the Leonard Cheshire Home, she was reluctant to make decisions and had definite opinions about her situation. She seemed to be saying that she was fine.

I felt that I had a duty to protect a client who was vulnerable and at risk of abuse. However, she was not mentally impaired and was an adult in charge of her own life. We had another case conference which included both Mr and Mrs B. Meanwhile the counsellor for the illness which afflicted Mrs B informed me that the situation was a classic example of a family with this disorder. I was aware that going to the Day Centre or challenging Mr B increased Mrs B's insecurity and she could not risk upsetting him.

I was finding the situation very difficult as I was under increasing pressure "to do something". I felt that both Mr and Mrs B were stuck in a situation that wasn't helping either of them. I felt that Mrs B was perhaps over-adapting – being grateful for any show of affection from her partner. Mr B I felt was doing nothing, burying his head in the sand but also perhaps becoming incapacitated. He had lost control over his son, he couldn't walk away from his wife and he could not cope with the role of carer.

After a long period of extremely difficult, threatening and emotionally draining circumstances, and careful monitoring, the multidisciplinary team were able to come to a satisfactory arrangement but not before the GP had given up and decided that Mrs B should be forcefully removed from the home for her own safety. We worked closely with all the family under this threat and gradually worked through the practical and emotional aspects of the situation. My focus was on Mrs B, others focused on the son and the father. Mr and Mrs B's son was beginning to care for his mother. He became hostile to other carers and they had to be withdrawn but gradually the son did become the formal carer for his mother, a totally unexpected outcome! Mrs B was very happy with this arrangement for a time but eventually other unexpected factors occurred that altered the situation. Mrs B's father and sister came and took her away to spend some time with them. Mr B does not have any further contact with his wife and son as far as I am aware."

This long and painful story illustrates some of the wider aspects of current structures and resource pools that are needed to contribute to collaborative care and ground-level practices. The pool includes practical and material resources, such as time and money, and a great deal of human resources in terms of emotional work, sustained commitment, dealing with uncertainty and anxiety and developing a helping relationship built on trust. Without the collaborative attention she received from many other faceworkers in the primary, secondary and participative meetings and conversations it is doubtful that this care manager would have had the successes she had, and the situation could have resulted in distress and failure.

Revisiting collaborative framework III: domain and faceworker functions

The situation described above captures many aspects of overlapping boundaries and the contributions of professions, agencies and faceworkers to shared tasks and activities. The domain of professional competence is taken as a given in the above scenario, including careful risk assessment and the management of complex, multi-user situations. A domain is described by Sally Hornby, as – 'the area in which a person or corporate body has power to function' (page 151). Agency domains often have geographical boundaries and may impose their own particular styles and methods of working. The boundaries of these domains may however overlap since in our society people are increasingly mobile. Achieving collaboration across these boundaries of responsibility, authority and role is not simple, but can be achieved if there is a willingness to focus on the needs of the users and carers and manage the complexities of inter-domain working.

The general domain of faceworkers is defined by their role and function. However, as the above extract illustrates, often the faceworker defines his or her own role, method of helping and overall function in negotiations with users. This aspect of collaboration is extended when the faceworker then negotiates clear areas of responsibility with other people in the situation in partnership with users, carers, and other individuals and agencies involved in the situation.

One interesting aspect of the story is the son who eventually negotiated a domain for himself as his mother's carer. This instance is an example of the points made by Sally Hornby in stressing the domain of informal helpers (page 153). It is also an example of unexpected consequences, the value of taking time, not being in a coercive frame of mind and sharing a willingness to tolerate uncertainty. Learning from instances, such as with various aspects of this case study, leads to the development of greater levels of collaboration, an internalisation of new ways of working and developing relationships. Mapping the communication patterns and new perspectives between agencies, faceworkers and different kinds of helpers appears to generate plans that can operate on a long-term basis and contribute to wider aspects of organisational learning.

Complex situations almost always provide a forum for consideration of many facets for users, not least those of addressing the needs of the wider family. They also provide for an exploration of many roles and functions. Collaboration in such situations requires a readiness to explore new ideas, new methods of practice and an open attitude to change. These new methods of practice may involve modifications of professional and agency roles, the ethos of helping organisations and the relative power positions of various helpers. Given the features and effects of change mentioned above it would not be surprising if some defensive behaviours, both individual and organisational, were to surface. Providing general role identity and security appears to be crucial for faceworkers to cope with their own potential for defensive behaviours, but there could also be a need for specific deliberate and skilled interventions to enable workers to confront their own fears and anxieties. Enabling faceworkers appears to be the best way of teaching them to enable others, whether those others are the users and carers who are the subject of their services, or peers and colleagues in multiprofessional, multi-agency teams all working towards improving their abilities to develop truly collaborative practice.

Conclusions to Part III

The aim of all services is to develop meaningful relations that enable users and carers to manage their own situations. In Part III it has been suggested that collaboration between faceworkers and those at the planning levels of health and social care organisations is equally important if these aims are to be achieved at ground-level practice.

The complexity of work at the ground level needs to be understood in terms of both material and human resources. Collaboration is an intensely human activity and it is suggested that the human resource element, as an input into the development of helping relationships, is often overlooked because of a failure to develop important levels of dialogue and communication. The case studies provide examples of unfolding stories, full of instances of emotional levels of work and the complexities of the operational levels of inter-professional, inter-agency working.

In line with Sally's earlier work, the team have revisited and explored role identity and security, both of which lie at the heart of the helping relationship. However, the roles of the user or carer and the faceworker can adapt under the confident and skilled application of their experience by senior faceworkers. Recognition that ambiguity and uncertainty are natural parts of this adaptation process is seen as crucial. Support, expressed in the forms of valuing, holding to rich patterns of dialogue and communication, and building faceworker-manager teams, must be forthcoming if collaborative practice is to be successful.

Glossary

This is a short list of selected conceptual terms with working definitions related specifically to the context of collaboration.

Anti-task When the primary task of an institution becomes implicitly redefined because it has become too difficult owing to societal, political or other pressures it becomes an anti-task.

Basic caring relationship The minimal essential relationship, based on respect and concern for another person.

Care Looking after, with human concern, through tending and protecting. Including an element of helping, and often used as a comprehensive term to cover both care and help.

Care-compact Methods of care, integrated to meet the needs of a particular user.

Carer The term includes:
   Informal carers personal carers – 'the carers'; local carers – friends and neighbours or local group volunteers; mutual helpers in a self-help group.
   formal carers Practitioners and other workers in the formal helping services.

Case conference/meeting That between faceworkers in the absence of the user.

Collaboration The comprehensive term to describe a relationship based on working together to achieve a common purpose. Types of collaboration are:
   Primary collaboration faceworker and user;
   Secondary collaboration faceworkers together;
   Participatory collaboration user and faceworkers together.
   Levels of collaboration include: routine or functional co-operation; simple; complex.

Compact 'A covenant; a structure; a composition. To join or knit firmly and tightly together; to make or compose. Compacted: firmly put together'.

Competence Capacity deriving from personal qualities, ability, experience and training. Spheres of competence include: field-competence; setting-competence; method-competence; function-competence.

214

Levels of competence include: basic competence; proficiency; expertness/specialisation.

Concurrent user An informal carer for whom help is also necessary.

Confection/to confect An organic process for making a whole by the mixture of constituents. Applied to helping, the particular blending and timing of either task-components to make up a work-task, or constituent tasks to make up an overall helping-task.

Confederacy 'A union by league or contract between persons, bodies of men, or states, for mutual support or joint action; an alliance, a compact'.

Confederate group Organised on a voluntary basis, having no built-in authority structure.

Co-operation Routine or functional collaboration.

Coping methods Ways which enable the faceworker to function optimally in stressful situations, without adverse after-effects. Including personal and professional coping mechanisms, informal and structured support.

Defence mechanisms Unrecognised processes serving to prevent a faceworker from experiencing role-insecurity in any situation. They may be personal, professional or institutional. They hinder collaboration.

Domain The area in which an individual or group has authority and power to function for a given purpose. It may be general or specific (applying in a particular case only), exclusive or overlapping.

Domain overlap/co-domain An area shared between more than one agency or faceworker.

Domain-mapping Defining individual responsibilities and work-tasks in relation to an overall helping-task.

Embedded power This term describes the informal and hidden seams of power that exist within institutions and are as potent as the formal structures and visible power distributions.

Empowerment Enabling a person or group to extend their sphere of activity and influence.

Enablement Non-specific intervention which actively engages users in finding solutions to their own troubles and helps them to help themselves.

Faceworker One who works at the interface with the user, including all formal and informal carers.

Fields of help Dependency – the young and the old – physical ill-health, mental ill-health, disability, social disadvantage and social maladjustment.

First-door methods Those that are appropriate to the user's first request for help.

Generalist practitioner One who has wide-ranging competence and/or has specialised in first-door methods.

Help Assistance in order to maintain or improve a situation. Including an element of caring and often used as a comprehensive term to cover both help and care.

Help-compact   Help-methods integrated to meet the needs of a particular user. It has duration and stages.

Help-method   A defined process, for providing care, treatment or enablement, developed to meet particular kinds of situation, and using institutional, organisational, material and human resources.

Helper   The all-embracing term including self-helpers as well as face-workers.

Helping approach   A standpoint, resulting from a particular interpretation of the general aim of helping (the well-being of the user).

Helping-task   The sum of human input necessary for carrying out a help-compact. It may be carried out by one helper or many. It may contain a number of task-components, and the overall task may contain many constituent or work-tasks.

Identity   sameness, sharing common qualities, being identical; having individuality, being unique.

Internal identity   that experienced by the individual or group.

External identity   that experienced by the individual or group and others.

Perceived identity   that experienced by others, coloured by their subjective reactions.

To identify   to make one with, to determine the identity of.

Identity-base   A group of workers with whom a faceworker feels at home.

Integrative approach   Derived from a view of the human being, as a unique physical, psychological and spiritual organism with a function and a place in society. It incorporates holistic, relational, family, community and collaborative approaches.

MEA – minimum essential assessment, as distinct from an 'extended assessment'.

MEC – minimum essential collaboration. Involvement of the minimal number of people, and the minimal amount of their time essential to the helping-task.

Mirroring process   The playing out by workers of the current relational patterns of a user.

Modelling   The provision by a faceworker of a model of behaviour which can be incorporated by a user or another faceworker.

Operational group   Designed for carrying out certain methods or functions, and having an in-built authority structure, usually with an operational leader.

Organisational learning   This occurs when something causes a change in the norms and culture that regulate the performance of an institution or organisation.

Para-helping organisations   Organisations of ordinary life, such as schools, churches and community groups, which can supplement the helping services.

Participatory conference/meeting   That between user and faceworkers.

Part-person identity   Based on core identity and certain aspects of extended identity, confected for the fulfilment of a particular role; often experienced as if it were the whole person.

Primary faceworker   The role of the helper with whom the user has the most important interface contact at any particular time.

Power-position   That of a person or group in relation to others. Often used, deliberately or unwittingly, to define the roles of others.

Practitioner province   The sphere of activity of a practitioner based on professional qualification, competence, experience and personal qualities. It is less than the professional province, since it includes only some of the extended competence of the profession. It may be greater than the practitioner's domain which is defined by a particular job description and its interpretation.

Professional province   The sphere of activity of a profession as a whole, delineated according to the fields, settings, methods and functions of help in which its members are competent to practice.
   Core province   competence belonging to every member;
   Extended province   competence belonging to certain members, through proficiency or specialisation in one of the fields of competence. External boundaries are defined in relation to those of users, other professions and groups of helpers, with which there may be a provincial overlap.

Projection   The belief that others share one's own subjective mental life. Individuals and groups may project unwanted characteristics of their own onto others in order to avoid having to deal with them.

Province   The sphere of activity of an individual or group of people, determined by competence. It may be exclusive or overlapping.

Provincial overlap/shared province   An area shared between two or more individuals or groups.

Repeating pattern   A relational pattern formed in childhood which is repeated in later life.

Resource pool   All the resources available to the residents of a particular locality: ordinary life resources; self-help organisations and groups; the informal carers; the helping services.

Role   A part to be fulfilled by an individual or a group, in respect of a task or in relation to another person or group.

Role-care   Looking after a particular role, including maintenance, development, promotion and protection.

Role-insecurity   Lack of self-confidence as a result of personal anxiety and/or uncertainty-in-role.

Sectional view   That provided by the profession or agency, from which the faceworker approaches a situation.

Self-helper One who helps him or herself, usually in collaboration with a faceworker or in a self-help group.

Sense-of-identity The experience of being oneself, to which the pronoun 'I' is ascribed. There is a fundamental need for a secure and satisfying sense-of-identity.

Separatism Use of the sectional view, to serve narrow sectional self-interest, rather than the needs of users.

System A structure with an internal organisation, designed to sustain itself and carry out its functions; with an external boundary which separates it from its environment and other systems, and creates an interface across which intake, output and relationships take place. It may contain sub-systems or be part of a supra-system.

Triple aim of helping The general aim of helping (well-being of the user) interpreted according to the integrated helping-approach: maximum self-responsibility; optimum quality of life; personal and social integration.

Trouble A comprehensive term to cover physical, emotional, mental, personal and social needs, problems, difficulties, disorders, disability, disadvantage and maladjustment. It may be the presenting, concurrent, underlying or target trouble.

Uncertainty-in-role A state in which the faceworkers are either: unsure of their working-identity or working-base; in an unduly stressful situation; or carrying the group uncertainty of a profession, agency or community group.

User An individual, family or small group (as distinct from a community group), having a trouble which causes them to seek help.

User-unit The user when composed of more than one person.

Viewing-point The position from which helpers look at a situation, determined by their personal and/or professional values, attitudes and training, it can take in a wide view or focus on a detail.

Working-base The position within an agency from which a working-role is carried out. It includes physical, organisational and psychological conditions.

Working-identity The identity of one in a working-role, to which is brought the individual's core-identity, aspects of extended identity, professional and agency and other group identifications, motivation and personal commitment.

Working-role That of an individual fulfilling a work-role and bringing to it something of their individual identity. The actor's interpretation of the scripted part.

Work-role A composite role incorporating the particular activities, responsibilities and formal relationships of a helper. Often defined in a job-description.

Work-task The task of a particular individual, when the overall helping-task is shared between a number of helpers.

Further Reading for Parts I and II

Capra, F. (1982) *The Turning Point*. Wildwood House and Fontana Paperbacks, London, esp. ch. 9.

Coleman, A.D. and Bexton, W.H. (1975) *Group Relations Reader*, Vol 1, Grex Sausalito, California.

Coleman, A.D. and Geller, M.H. (1985) *Group Relations Reader*, Vol II, Goetz Printing, Springfield, Virginia.

Douglas, T. (1978) *Basic Groupwork*. Tavistock Publications, London.

Grotstein, J.S. (1985) Splitting and Projective Identification. Jason Aronson, New Jersey and London.

Hinchelwood, R. (1987) *What Happens in Groups*. Free Association Books, London.

Lawrence, W. (ed.) (1989) *Exploring Individual and Organisational Boundaries*. John Wiley, Chichester.

Mattinson, J. (1975) The Reflection Process in Casework Supervision. Tavistock Publications, London.

Menzies Lyth, I. (1988) *Containing Anxiety in Institutions*. Free Association Books, London.

Schon, D. (1988) *Educating the Reflective Practitioner*. Jossey-Bass Publishers, San Francisco and London.

Skynner, R. (1989) *Institutions and How to Survive Them*. Methuen, London.

Stevens, A. (1982) *Archetype*. Routledge and Kegan Paul, London.

Woodhouse, D. & Pengelly, P. (1991) *Anxiety and the Dynamics of Collaboration*. Aberdeen University Press, Aberdeen.

Users and Carers

Becker, S. & Aldridge, J. (1993) *Children Who Care: Inside the World of Young Carers*. Loughborough University.

Pitkeathley, J. (1989) *It's My Duty, Isn't It? The Plight of Carers*. Souvenir Press, London.

Richardson, A., Unell, J., & Aston, B. (1989) *A New Deal for Carers*. King's Fund Centre, London.

School of Advanced Urban Studies, Bristol, (1993) Study No 7. 'Working together for better community care'.

Nursing
Contributed by Patricia Webb, RGN, Dip, Soc. Res., RCNT, Lecturer, Trinity Hospice, London.

Calman, J. (1983) *Talking with Patients*. Heinemann, London.
Calman, M. (1987) *Health and Illness – the Lay Perspective*. Tavistock Publications, London.
Egan, G. (1985) *The Skilled Helper*. Brooks Cole Publishing, Pacific Grove, California.
Jensen, U.J. & Morley, G. (1990) *Changing Values in Medical and Health Carer Decision-Making*. John Wiley, Chichester.
Ley, P. (1988) *Communicating with Patients*. Croom Helm, London.
Maxwell, R. & Weaver, W. (eds) (1984) *Public Participation in Health*. King Edward's Hospital Fund for London.
Niven, N. (1989) *Health Psychology*. Churchill Livingstone, Edinburgh.
Stoll, B.A. (1989) *Ethical Dilemmas in Cancer Care*. Macmillan, London.

General medical practice
Contributed by Judy Shakespeare, MA, BM, BCh, MRCP, MRCGP, General Practitioner.

Balint, M. (1964) *The Doctor, his Patient and the Illness*. Churchill Livingstone, Edinburgh.
Blane, D. (1986) 'Health professionals' in *Sociology as Applied to Medicine*. Patrick, D. (ed.) 2nd edn., Baillière Tindall, London.
Freeling, P. & Harris, C.M. (1984) *The Doctor Patient Relationship*. 3rd edn, Churchill Livingstone, Edinburgh.
Gregson, B., Carlidge, A. & Bond, J. (1991) 'Interprofessional collaboration in primary health care organisations'. Occasional Paper 52. Royal College of General Practitioners, London.
Jones, R.V.H. (1986) 'Working together – learning together'. Occasional paper 33. Royal College of General Practitioners, London.
Neighbour, R. (1987) *The Inner Consultation*. Kluwer Academic Publishers, Netherlands.
Pritchard, P. & Pritchard, J. (1992) *Developing Primary Teamwork in Primary Health Care. A Practical Workbook*. Practical Guides for General Practice No. 15. Oxford Medical Publications, Oxford.

Social work
Contributed by David Howe, BSc, MA, PhD Senior Lecturer in Social Work, University of East Anglia.

Ballett, C. & Birchall, E. (1992) *Co-ordination in Child Protection – a Review of the Literature.* HMSO, London.

Bayley, M., Seyd, R. & Tennant, A. (1989) *Local Health and Welfare: Is Partnership Possible?.* Gower, Aldershot.

Charles, M. with Stevenson, O. (1990) Multidisciplinary is different! Child Protection: Working Together. University of Nottingham.

Darvill, G. & Smale, G. (Eds.) (1990) *Partners in Empowerment.* Volume II: *Networks of Innovation in Social Work.* (Ed. G. Darvill, 1990) National Institute for Social Work, London.

Hey, A, Minty, B. & Trowell, J. (1991) 'Inter-professional and inter-agency work: theory, practice and training for the nineties', in: Pietroni, M. (ed.) *Right or Privilege? Post Qualifying Training for Social Workers with Special Reference to Child Care.* CCETSW Study 10, Central Council for Education and Training of Social Workers, London.

HMSO, (1990) *Caring for People: Community Care in the Next Decade.* HMSO, London.

Stevenson, O. & Hallett, C. (1980) *Child Abuse: Aspects of Interprofessional Co-operation.* Allen & Unwin, London.

Journals

British Journal of General Practice
Thomas, R.V.R. & Corney, R.H. (1992) 'A survey of links between mental health professionals and general practice in six district health authorities'. **42**(362): 358–61.

British Journal of Social Work
Bourne, P., Evans, R. & Tattersall, A. (1993) 'Stress and coping in social workers: a preliminary investigation'. Vol. 23.

Webb, A., Vincent, J., Wistow, G. & Wray, K. (1991) 'Developmental social care: experimental community mental handicap teams in Nottinghamshire'. Vol. 21.

British Medical Journal
Ashley-Miller, M. (1990) 'Community care'. **300**(6723): 487.

Pietroni, P. (1992) 'Beyond the boundaries: relationship between general practice and complementary medicine'. **305**(6853): 564–6.

Health & Social Care in the Community
McIntosh, J. & Bennett-Emslie, G. (1993) 'The health centre as a location for care management'. **1**(2), 91–7.

Journal of Advanced Nursing
Iles, P.A. & Auluck, R. (1990) 'From organisational to interorganisational development in working practice: improving the effectiveness of interdisciplinary teamwork and interagency collaboration'. **15**(1), 50–58.

Journal of Interprofessional Care
Ash, E. (1992) 'The personal-professional interface in learning: towards reflective education. **6**(3), 261–72.
Biggs, S. (1993) 'User participation and interprofessional collaboration in community care.' **7**(2), 151–60.
Hutchinson, A. & Gordon, S. (1992) 'Primary care teamwork – making it a reality'. **6**(1), 31–42.

Journal of Medical Ethics
Wilson-Barnett, J. (1989) 'Limited authority and partnership: professional relationships in health care'. **15**: 12–16.

Journal of Social Work Practice
Cooper, A. (1992) 'Anxiety and child protection work in two national systems', **6**(2).
Hornby, S. (1983) 'Collaboration in social work: a major practice issue'. **1**(1).

References for Part III

Bain, A. (1982) *The Baric Experiment: The Design of Jobs and Organi-sation for the Expression and Growth of Human Capacity.* Tavistock Institute of Human Relations Occasional Paper no. 4.

Baker, R., Hearnshaw, H., and Robertson, N. (1999) *Implementing Change with Clinical Audit.* Wiley, Chichester.

Buchanan, D. and Badman, R. (1999) *Power, Politics and Organisational Change.* Sage, London.

Dechant, K., Marsick. V.J., and Kasi, E. (1993) Towards a model of team learning. *Studies in Continuing Education,* **15** 1–14

Gillett, A.M. (1995) Future challenges of the social services in the building of the European welfare society. *Journades Internacionales de Surveis Sociales,* Barcelona, Generalitat de Catalunya Benstar Social, pp. 355–60.

Finlay, L. (2000) The challenge of working in teams *in* A. Brechin, H. Brown and M. Eby (eds), *Critical Practice in Health and Social Care.* Sage, London.

Hudson, B. (2000) Inter-agency collaboration – a sceptical view *in* A. Brechin, H. Brown, and M. Eby (eds). *Critical Practice in Health and Social Care.* Sage, London.

James, J. and Dewhurst, J. (1995) Death in Service. *Health Service Journal,* 18 May, 26.

Khaleelee, O. and Miller. J. (1985) *From Dependence to Autonomy.* Free Association Books, London.

Laungani, P. and Williams, G.A. (1997) Patient-focused care: effects of organisational change on the stress of community health professionals. *International Journal of Health Education,* Vol. 35, No.4, pp.108–114.

Lucas, B., Harrison-Read, P., Tyrer, P. and Rapp, D. (1997) Falling through the net: discrepancies between mental health services in care plans and patients recently discharged from a community mental health team. *Journal of Interprofessional Care,* Vol. 11, No. 3, pp. 303–311.

Marris, P. (1986) *Loss and Change.* Routledge, London.

McCrea, C. (1999) Good clinical audit requires teamwork, *in* R. Baker, H.

Hearnshaw and N. Robertson, (eds) *Implementing Change in Clinical Audit*. Wiley, Chichester.

Menzies-Lyth, I. (1998) *Containing Anxiety in Institutions*. Free Association Books, London.

Muir-Grey, J.A. (1998) *Evidence-based Policy Making*. Churchill Livingstone, London.

NHS Executive (1997) *Clinical Governance: Quality in the new NHS*. HMSO, London.

Schein, E.H. (1988) *Organisational Psychology*. Prentice-Hall, Englewood-Cliffs, NJ.

Secretary of State (1997) *The New NHS Modern – Dependable*. HMSO, London.

Senge, P. (1990) *The Fifth Discipline: the Art and Practice of the Learning Organisation*. Doubleday, New York.

Strauss, A., Schatzman, L., Erlich, D., Bucher, R., and Sabshin, M. (1973) The hospital and its negotiated order *in* G. Salaman and K. Thomson (eds), *People and Organisations*. Longman, London.

Teram, E. (1997) Interprofessional teams as a form of organisational control, unpublished thesis. Wilfred Laurier University, Faculty of Social Work, Waterloo, Ontario, Canada.

Tushman, M.L. (1977) A political approach to organisations: a review and rationale, *Academy of Management Review,* Vol. 2, No. 2.

Index